Autism, Asperger's & ADHD

WHAT YOU NEED TO KNOW

A Guide for Parents, Students and other Professionals

SIMON BIGNELL

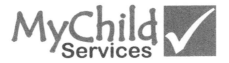

First Printing, 2018

Bignell, Simon.

Autism, Asperger's & ADHD: What You Need to Know. *A Guide for Parents, Students and other Professionals* / Simon Bignell

ISBN 978-1-9996667-0-5 (pbk.)
ISBN 978-1-9996667-1-2 (ebk.)

Printed in Great Britain.

MyChild Services Publishing is a Division of MyChild Services Ltd. Registered Office: Coppice Side Venture Park, North Street, Nottingham, Nottinghamshire, UK, NG16 4DF.
www.MyChildServices.com

Links to third party websites are provided by MyChild Services Publishing in good faith and for information only.

A catalogue record for this book is available from the British Library.

You can cite this book by using the following APA reference:

Bignell, S. (2018). *Autism, Asperger's & ADHD: What You Need to Know. A Guide for Parents, Students and other Professionals.* Nottingham: MyChild Services Publishing.

For Fatima, Bessie and Bertie.

With all my love.

About the Author

Simon Bignell PhD, SFHEA, MBPsS, CPsychol

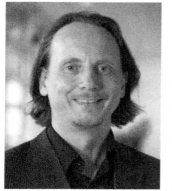 Dr Simon Bignell is a Senior Lecturer in Psychology at the University of Derby, a Senior Fellow of the Higher Education Academy and a published author on children's developmental conditions. He specialises in Autism and ADHD and has a PhD in ADHD and children's language from the University of Essex.

He is the author of the final-year undergraduate course 'Autism, Asperger's & ADHD', which he has taught since 2006, and has been studied by over 25,000 learners. He is qualified in the TEACCH Autism program and has supported children and young adults with autism and ADHD and their families for many years in academic and voluntary work. He has been awarded research grants, published in scientific books, journals and encyclopaedias and has given invited keynote talks at conferences around the world.

With his wife, Dr Fatima Bignell, a Local Authority Educational Psychologist, he is the Co-Director of MyChild Services Ltd (www.mychildservices.com), a company that provides Educational Psychology support for children with Special Educational Needs for parents, Local Authorities, Schools and Academies. They live in Derbyshire in the UK with their two young children.

www.SimonBignell.com

Contents

Preface

This book summarises the essential information on the spectrum of autism and Attention-Deficit/Hyperactivity Disorder (ADHD) so that you do not have to go looking for it when straight answers are needed about the real-world issues facing people with these conditions and their families. I have written this book to be a no-nonsense guide that draws from research and practical experience and summarises essential things that every person should know about the autism spectrum and ADHD.

In addition to the body of scientific work from which this book draws, the words here are the result of my work with people who have these conditions. They are also a product of the many hundreds of lectures I have given, visits to schools I have made, and the conversations with parents, teachers and students that I have had over the last 20 years. I have kept the weighty academic theory, which often accompanies such descriptions, to the fundamentals to appeal to a broader readership.

The book does not attempt to give an insight into what it is like to have autism or ADHD, as I believe that should come from people with these conditions. However, the voices of people with these conditions, their families and their experiences across a variety of settings has heavily informed the content.

The themes highlighted across these chapters are supported by a large body of scientific investigation including my own published research within Developmental Psychology. In an age of misinformation and *fake news*, this evidence-based approach is necessary, as the way we think about these conditions, and the way we try to help people with them is continually changing. I hope that this book will be of value for many years to come to parents, professionals and students seeking to understand further and increase sensitivity to these fascinating conditions.

In support of the community surrounding people with these conditions, in parallel to this book I have written a 100% free online course (MOOC) 'Understanding Autism, Asperger's & ADHD' with University of Derby Online. This course, which is endorsed by The ADHD Foundation, features many video case studies, interviews and multimedia content www.derby.ac.uk/online/free-courses. I have also written two short courses to extend knowledge of autism for Parents and Educational Professionals.

If you would like to consider taking part in research studies about autism and ADHD, please visit **www.ASDresearch.org** to register your interest. You can also subscribe to our Newsletter to be kept up to date with the latest research studies, Local Authority policy, teaching practice and parenting advice from all the most current sources.

Dr Simon Bignell

May 2018

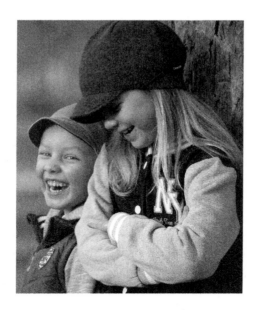

Chapter 1 – Introduction

This book is organised to help you learn about these complex and fascinating conditions. The chapters map loosely to my 'Autism, Asperger's and ADHD' final-year undergraduate course that I have taught at the University of Derby in the UK since 2006. Since then, thousands of learners have taken the course, and many students have gone on to apply this knowledge directly in the field. For many learners, this knowledge has helped them to understand better the people they work with, their friends and family. For some learners who have taken this course, it has opened the doorway to their understanding of themselves and been the catalyst for their diagnosis. For others, who have this information, it has helped them to care for their children or to teach their pupils more effectively.

The conditions covered in this book and the themes throughout are 'hot topics' and can act as a trigger to anxiety and provoke strong reactions in some people. These sensitivities are sometimes a result of a positive movement to reclaim, from Psychiatry and Psychology, the way the public perceives and treats people with autism and ADHD. It is understandable and correct that autistic people and those diagnosed with ADHD may view these differences from others as fundamental to their identity and want to protect the integrity of such on their terms.

The growing appreciation from inside and outside the fields of Psychiatry and Psychology that the voice of the 'patient' is ultimately more important than that of the practitioner is a sign of the times and encouraging. For too long, misunderstanding and misinformation have existed between authorities and people in their care. These sensitivities must be acknowledged if lasting progress is to be made scientifically and socially. The mistrust of medical and professional authority has been frustrated by the ever-changing diagnostic standards and descriptions adopted by the psychiatric and medical manuals that determine under what conditions a person has a particular 'disorder' or 'illness'. It is vital to bridge the divide between people who may need support and people who commit their lives to providing it.

Today, opinions are divided on the validity of the *medical model* of illness and its appropriateness to conditions such as the autism spectrum and ADHD. Sensitivities of talking about the autism spectrum and ADHD from the person, parent and practitioner perspective are respectfully considered throughout this book. Although the convention is to use person-first language (e.g. 'a person with ADHD'; 'a person with autism', etc.), this has been used variously with other ways of referring to people (e.g. 'autistic', etc.). This usage is in keeping with recent opinion surveys of how some groups of people wish to be referred. I hope the text here respects the uniqueness and individuality of those described throughout.

The Great Need for Autism and ADHD Understanding

Autism Spectrum Disorder

As it is often said, *"If you know one person with autism, then you know one person with autism"*. It is possible to generalise about autism, but it is important to realise that each person's type of autism varies, as does the extent to which the symptoms are problematic for them. Many of the problems faced by autistics are because they live in a world that is not conducive to their unique differences and sometimes not accepting.

There is a great need for further understanding of autism in the general public. A recent study by the National Autistic Society (NAS) showed that while most people have heard of autism, very few show a detailed understanding of it. This lack of understanding of the needs of autistic people and their families was the focus of a recent NAS 'Too Much Information' campaign, which sought to challenge the myths, misconceptions and stereotypes that can make autistic people feel so isolated and can make society feel so unwelcoming for them.

A landmark Parliamentary debate on autism was held in 2016 by the 'All-Party Parliamentary Group on Autism' at the House of Commons in the UK, chaired by the Member of Parliament Mrs Cheryl Gillan. The purpose of this influential group of politicians was:

> "To raise awareness of issues affecting people with autism and Asperger syndrome, their families and carers; to raise Parliamentary awareness of autism; to campaign for changes to government policy to benefit people with autism and Asperger syndrome and improve diagnosis or support for people with autism and Asperger syndrome".

> ('World Autism Awareness Week - Hansard Online', n.d.)

They concluded that people with autism are highly valuable to society and although there is good public awareness of autism, there is a great need for public autism understanding. They found that just 15 percent of adults on the autism spectrum are in full-time paid work, and across the country there exist insufficient services for people with autism and their

3

families. There is an urgent need to improve waiting times for diagnosis and low-cost, evidence-based services.

Data from the United States suggests that autism is financially costly, costing upwards of $35 billion each year in direct (both medical and non-medical) and indirect costs to care for all people diagnosed with autism (Ganz, M.L. cited in Moldin & Rubenstein, 2006). When costs are projected across the lifespan, the incremental societal cost is estimated at $3.2 million for every person with autism. Lost productivity and adult care are the most significant components of the costs (Ganz, 2007).

It is not known what the current financial cost of autism is, but irrespective of the financial costs there is a strong argument to provide evidence-based early interventions and support for people with autism (both those diagnosed and those not) and for their families and carers. Increasing awareness of autism is slowly being reflected in Government policy and accordingly in practice through service provision and in public attitudes and understanding of the condition.

Attention-Deficit/Hyperactivity Disorder

Attention-Deficit/Hyperactivity Disorder (ADHD), like autism, is a complex condition and the task of trying to understand it fully and other conditions that are usually first diagnosed in childhood is not straightforward. In the first chapter, we will build on our existing understanding of ADHD: we will explore how common it is, how the symptoms relate to having a diagnosis of the condition and the consequences for people of having ADHD across the lifespan.

When considering conditions such as ADHD, it helps to think about what it might feel like for the person. Try to think about what other clinical conditions might be present at the same time and how these may interact with each other. For example, if a person is also affected by Anxiety or

Depression, this may significantly change the way their ADHD presents to those around them. After finding out more about ADHD, you will notice that the condition rarely presents on its own and is usually accompanied by several other conditions, many of which may go undiagnosed and untreated. Over time people with ADHD report the way that their symptoms manifest changes, they tend to adapt and grow into their ADHD and learn ways to cope; this can sometimes mean that a diagnosis is no longer appropriate in adulthood. ADHD in adults can look very different from when it characteristically initially appears in childhood.

In looking at ADHD, you should aim to place the person with the condition first and to try to understand the condition through their descriptions and experiences as far as possible. A shift in thinking may occur from understanding ADHD as a disruptive behavioural condition of childhood to one that affects people of all ages across a continuum of severity and, like autism, a spectrum of different characteristics.

When you hear about all the *markers* (symptoms) of autism and ADHD and the close relationship to other conditions, you may notice these types of behaviours and traits in someone you know, perhaps a family member or even in yourself. This does not indicate that you have an undiagnosed condition. However, if you do suspect that you or your child or someone you care for could benefit from support, it is important to seek more information and guidance. A good place to start is often your local General Practitioner who, if needed, can refer on to a specialist practitioner or clinic for assessment.

We will look at ADHD and Hyperkinetic Disorder in more detail in Chapter 2.

Resources

For more information about autism, visit the National Autistic Society (NAS) at their website:

www.autism.org.uk.

For more information about ADHD and related conditions, visit the ADHD Foundation at their website:

www.adhdfoundation.org.uk.

The National Institute for Health and Care Excellence (NICE) provides high-quality, evidence-based information to practitioners about autism and ADHD on their website:

Autism - www.nice.org.uk/guidance/qs51.

ADHD - www.nice.org.uk/guidance/qs39.

The Independent Parental Special Education Advice (IPSEA) charity offer free and independent legally based information, advice and support to help get the right education for children and young people with all kinds of special educational needs (SEN) and disabilities.

www.ipsea.org.uk.

If you would like to consider taking part in research studies about autism and ADHD, please visit www.ASDresearch.org to register your interest.

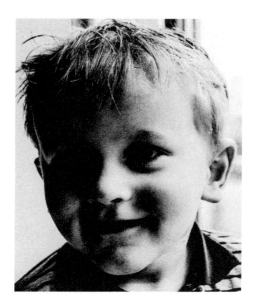

Chapter 2 – ADHD and Hyperkinetic Disorder

When you have studied this chapter, you will understand and be able to describe the main symptoms, subtypes and diagnostic criteria for ADHD and Hyperkinetic Disorder.

Key Points

- ADHD was described first over 100 years ago.
- It involves problems with attention, hyperactivity and impulsivity.
- It exists on a continuum of severity.
- Estimated prevalence rates vary considerably across research studies.
- Boys are more likely to be referred for help than girls are.
- ADHD usually occurs alongside other conditions.

What is Attention-Deficit/Hyperactivity Disorder?

ADHD is a common developmental disorder that affects thinking and behaviour due to underlying problems of poor attention, hyperactivity and impulsivity, and is linked to long-term adverse consequences. The exact causes of ADHD are not fully known, and there are likely to be multiple causes and complex interactions with other conditions. ADHD usually occurs alongside other conditions, and for some people affects them significantly throughout their lifetime.

Diagnostically the condition involves problems with attention, hyperactivity and impulsivity on a continuum of severity, usually being diagnosed in early childhood. Although some people are mostly affected by problems with hyperactivity and impulsivity, more often it occurs in those who show a mainly inattentive form. However, the profile in individuals that is by far the most frequently referred for help is where the core symptoms cluster together into a combined form of all three of the clinical markers.

ADHD is generally reported at about 6–7 percent of school-age children worldwide (Willcutt, 2012); although there is significant variability in the published prevalence rates worldwide, with the highest rates of referral, diagnosis and treatment reported in the USA. However, it is unclear if the underlying rates of ADHD, either diagnosed or undiagnosed, differ across countries, socioeconomic status or ethnicity. Parent-reported rates of ADHD in the UK are commonly lower than in the USA; one study shows around 1.4 percent of all school-age having a diagnosis (Russell, Rodgers, Ukoumunne, & Ford, 2014). Boys are much more likely to be referred for clinical assessment of the condition than girls are.

The condition is commonly credited as being first identified well over 100 years ago by Sir George Frederick Still, who is sometimes known as the *father* of British paediatrics. He was one of the country's first professors of child medicine and gave early descriptions of children that had problems with maintaining their attention, who were often aggressive, defiant and resistant to discipline but with normal levels of intelligence. In the years since those early descriptions, science has come to refine what we know about the condition, and definitions and names have been modified to reflect this increase in knowledge about ADHD.

The idea of unrestrained behaviour as a medical problem has its origins in eighteenth- and nineteenth-century early accounts of children who presented behaviour resembling modern-day ADHD. In his historical account of ADHD, Eric Taylor (2011) traces Still's 'Disorders of Moral Control' through to modern-day Hyperkinetic Disorder and raises critical cultural issues about how far control was, and still is, expected of children.

In recent years, there has been a resolution over what we might name this group of commonly occurring symptoms. For example, in the past, the same condition has variously been known as 'Minimal Brain Dysfunction', 'Hyperkinetic Syndrome', and 'Attention-Deficit Disorder' – a term that is still used in North America but seems to refer less to the hyperactive-impulsive nature of the condition. Likewise, the term 'hyperactivity' is often used in everyday conversations to describe intense or overexcited children.

Hyperkinetic Disorder

The term 'Hyperkinetic Disorder' is employed in the World Health Organization's diagnostic manual, the *International Statistical Classification of Diseases and Related Health Problems*, (10th rev.; ICD– 10; World Health Organization, 1992) to refer to a similar condition to ADHD. This term is often used interchangeably within the UK's National Health Service (NHS) literature, along with the more frequently used term Attention-Deficit/Hyperactivity Disorder. ADHD is the term defined in the *Diagnostic and Statistical Manual of Mental Disorders*, (5th ed.; DSM–5;

American Psychiatric Association, 2013) and is also the term most frequently used in research studies.

Diagnoses of ADHD and Hyperkinetic Disorder are based on a similar set of symptoms across inattention, hyperactivity and impulsivity. The main difference for Hyperkinetic Disorder is that the diagnostic criteria in the ICD diagnostic manual require all three of the core indicators to be present, whereas, for ADHD, these are grouped into subtypes. The ICD manual uses a narrower diagnostic category, which includes people with more-severe symptoms and impairment.

The Symptoms of ADHD

The various terms used for ADHD can be confusing; they mostly describe the problems of children who are hyperactive and have difficulty concentrating. The core indications of ADHD are usually described as threefold: poor attention, hyperactivity and impulsivity, with the last two often being grouped in research and for classification purposes. The reality is that hyperactivity and impulsivity, although different entities when precisely defined, are practically very hard behaviours to separate from one another.

Not all children with ADHD have all the symptoms; for example, some children are affected by inattention more than they are by hyperactivity and impulsivity. For a diagnosis to be made several symptoms must be present before the age of 12 years. Within diagnostic practice, this clustering of core markers into categories generates three possible diagnostic subtypes of ADHD:

i) 'Predominantly Hyperactive-Impulsive type'.
ii) 'Predominantly Inattentive type'.
iii) 'Combined type' ADHD.

Combined-type is the most frequently diagnosed subtype of ADHD. In the most recent version of the diagnostic manual (DSM-5) 'presentation specifiers' have replaced these subtypes, but they map directly on to one another and most previously diagnosed children have been allocated to one of these categories. Historically, some children have received a 'Not Otherwise Specified' (NOS) category that allows a diagnosis but where the full number of symptoms are not reached.

At the core, ADHD is a cluster of difficulties with attention (or inattention), hyperactivity and impulsivity that are severe enough to cause problems throughout all parts of a person's life. These behaviours include difficulties such as a failure to pay close attention to detail, difficulty organising tasks and actions, excessive talking, fidgeting, or an inability to remain still in appropriate situations.

Here is a classic definition:

> "ADHD is a developmental disability with a childhood onset that typically results in a chronic and pervasive pattern of impairment in school, social and/or work domains and often in daily adaptive domains."

> (Goldstein & Ellison, 2002, p. 90).

This definition is both useful from a clinical and treatment perspective and in appreciating the diagnostic criteria for ADHD. However, ADHD is much more than these 'primary symptoms' and involves the child's ability to control their behaviour and to keep future goals and consequences in mind (Barkley, 2013). Over recent years, ADHD has been characterised increasingly in terms of neurology and executive function, with increased recognition of the delay in children's development rather than as a behavioural impairment.

Most typically developing children do at times show signs of over-activity, excitability, hyperactivity, inattention and lapses in focus or concentration. However, the defining feature of a child with ADHD is that these symptoms are severe, unremitting and present wherever he or she finds themselves (i.e. at school, at home or in the playground).

If the markers of ADHD are not present across multiple situations and persistent, then the clinician or Paediatrician may seek other explanations for these problematic behaviours, perhaps trying to explore why symptoms exist and what causes them. For example, there could be the presence of Anxiety, Oppositional Defiant Disorder or Conduct Disorder, which can sometimes resemble ADHD. If another clinical diagnosis could better explain the presence of symptoms, the clinician will also explore that possibility with appropriate assessments and will work within existing guidelines suitable for that suspected condition.

Children who show the signs of ADHD are often first brought to the attention of their school Special Educational Needs system, not because of their problematic behaviour, but because of their educational immaturity. Sometimes there is a delay in expressive or receptive language that becomes apparent when they first start primary school.

It is common to receive a diagnosis of ADHD at around the age of seven years when mixing with other children at school provides a natural comparison, and there is often for the first time a strong focus on educational ability and achievement. The school's Special Educational Needs (and Disability) Co-ordinator (SENCo/SENDCo) will usually be involved in identifying and organising support for children with additional educational needs. Educational assessments consider a child's strengths and difficulties, and standardised tests may be given to establish their ability and achievement levels compared to average scores of children of the same age.

The two core characteristics of ADHD (inattention and hyperactivity-impulsivity) are significantly different. One way of viewing the child's hyperactivity and impulsivity is at the behavioural level, as this is most apparent and often disruptive. Conversely, the inattentive symptoms can be considered at the executive (managerial) level of thoughts and the sequencing of information as the child cognitively filters, holds on to and processes information. There is a distinction between the types of symptoms seen in ADHD that are directly observable and those at the cognitive level. Functionally, these two levels of consideration interact with each other and are difficult to distinguish, presenting a challenge for researchers. Next, we will look in more detail at the core markers of ADHD and how these symptoms can manifest in children.

Inattention

Inattentiveness is a central characteristic of ADHD and is one of the clinical markers for diagnosis. Failure to pay close attention to detail or making careless mistakes when doing schoolwork or other activities and trouble with keeping attention focused during play or schoolwork is reported in people with the condition. Likewise, appearing not to listen when spoken to and failing to follow instructions or finish tasks can cause problems at school and home. These traits are likely to lead the person with ADHD to avoid tasks that require a high amount of mental effort and organisation, such as school projects or chores around the home. For example, a child with ADHD may frequently lose their schoolbooks or toys, be excessively distractible and be forgetful.

Other markers of ADHD may include procrastination and difficulty with beginning or completing activities. Practical problems may present, like problems with household activities, or there may be trouble falling asleep due to too many thoughts at night. These symptoms of ADHD can lead a child to frequent emotional outbursts, and frustration can result.

Hyperactivity-Impulsive Behaviour

Frustrating to a child with ADHD are the consequences of hyperactivity and impulsivity. Children with these traits are often 'on the go' and can have poor self-monitored behaviour. They often find it hard to settle down to a task; they are restless, fidgety, and always up and out of their seats. These children are impatient, talk frequently and have difficulty in delaying responses. Behaviours such as fidgeting with hands or feet or squirming in their seats and often leaving their seats can cause problems for the children in the school classroom. Equally, running or climbing at inappropriate times and difficulty maintaining quiet play can lead the children to feel restless. They may have excessive speech and answer questions before the speaker has finished. Other characteristics, such as failing to wait for their turn and interrupting the activities of others at inappropriate times, are often present. In adult life, these traits can present as negative behaviours such as impulsive spending, leading to financial difficulties.

Consequences of ADHD

The core symptoms of inattention, hyperactivity and impulsivity can lead to a vast number of negative consequences that combined can influence development and educational attainment such that some researchers have characterised this as a 'developmental lag'. In adulthood, the effects of ADHD can be considerable, leading to disorganisation, failed relationships and impulsive decision-making.

It is easy to focus on the less-desirable elements of ADHD without appreciating those that are positive. The child with boisterous hyperactivity and impulsive behaviour that was so troublesome in the rigidly disciplined setting of school, with time and increasing autonomy, may come to be an extroverted, outgoing person, often channelling the 'over-activity' into occupations or sports where these qualities are valued. Individuals with ADHD often have a tenacious and spontaneous character, which can be an asset under some circumstances.

Prevalence of ADHD

ADHD is one of the most common childhood conditions, about 2–5 percent of school-age children in the UK are thought to be diagnosed. In the USA it is reported that 8.4 percent of children have a current diagnosis of ADHD (Danielson et al., 2018). However, it is difficult to specify precisely how many children have been diagnosed with ADHD, as prevalence estimates vary significantly within the published reports and there is no reliable central database to which we can refer. Many studies have identified significant variability in ADHD prevalence estimates worldwide.

The perception that rates of ADHD diagnosis and treatment throughout the past few decades have increased has fuelled concerns about whether the actual prevalence of the condition has increased over time. According to the most comprehensive review of ADHD prevalence studies to date (Polanczyk, Willcutt, Salum, Kieling, & Rohde, 2014), there has been no evidence to suggest an increase over recent years in the number of children who meet criteria for ADHD when standardised diagnostic procedures are followed. They showed that variation in reported rates of diagnosis and treatment of ADHD were likely a reflection of increasing public awareness, access to treatment and changing clinical practices.

Gender Differences in ADHD

It is reported that males show higher rates of ADHD than females (Arnett, Pennington, Willcutt, DeFries, & Olson, 2015). Boys are up to six times more likely to be referred for assessment than girls are. However, this may be due to males' behaviour being expressed in a more visible, aggressive and troublesome way. An exact ratio of these traits may be closer to about three boys to every one girl.

Proportionally, girls are more frequently diagnosed with the inattentive form of ADHD than boys are, although this does not mean that all girls have the inattentive subtype and all boys have the hyperactive-impulsive subtype. It is also likely that the symptoms of ADHD go unnoticed more often in females than in males and fail to be referred for professional assessment. Boys tend to be more disruptive and attract more attention, whereas girls generally may be less obviously affected and present their symptoms more silently.

Conditions that often occur with ADHD

Parents of children with ADHD typically report that the most troublesome elements of having ADHD are not the primary symptoms but the secondary symptoms or those caused by other conditions that go alongside ADHD. Co-occurring disruptive behaviour, mood disorder, anxiety and substance abuse frequently accompany ADHD (Wilens & Spencer, 2010). However, the two most commonly occurring comorbid disorders are Oppositional Defiant Disorder and Conduct Disorder. These behavioural conditions account for many of the most problematic behavioural difficulties associated with ADHD.

One less obvious problem related to childhood ADHD is the associated difficulties with language skills that may accompany the condition. Children with ADHD frequently experience pragmatic language deficits, such as difficulties with their comprehension of figurative or non-literal language. Some children with ADHD have trouble making meaning from context, understanding figurative language, or understanding the dual meanings used in sarcasm and jokes. These difficulties seem to be most prevalent in children who show high levels of inattentiveness; even in non-diagnosed samples of children poor attention and elevated levels of hyperactivity often occur alongside pragmatic language weaknesses (Bignell & Cain, 2007). Likewise, the reading comprehension problems of children with attention difficulties are related to weak word reading, and listening comprehension is particularly vulnerable in children at risk of

ADHD (Cain & Bignell, 2014).

The frequent behavioural problems that are associated with ADHD may have a subsequent impact on children's cognitive, behavioural, emotional and academic performance, confounding the difficulties that these children can face. It is important to note that having a diagnosis of ADHD itself does not lead to a child misbehaving or being anti-social. However, conditions that frequently accompany ADHD, such as Oppositional Defiant Disorder and Conduct Disorder, may cause significant difficulties for the child. These behaviours, in school-age children, are characterised by talking back to adults, rejection by peers and failure in school. However, children with ADHD without these associated conditions who are followed into adolescence have been found only in some cases to exhibit anti-social behaviours into adolescence and adulthood (Ahmadi-Kashani & Hechtman, 2014).

The existence of other conditions alongside ADHD does not mean that one causes the other, but they may well make things worse. For example, having a short attention span and anxiety can lead to behaviours that are prone to misinterpretation by others, causing additional problems. Being always 'up and on the go' coupled with social and communication problems can lead a child to be misinterpreted by others as being deliberately disrespectful of personal boundaries or authority.

We will cover in more detail in Chapter 6 issues of comorbidity and related conditions that commonly exist alongside ADHD. However, it is important to realise that this condition rarely presents on its own.

Causes of ADHD

ADHD is among the most well studied of all childhood psychological disorders, and yet the causes of ADHD are not entirely known. ADHD is not caused by poor parenting or moral failure on the part of the child. In the last few decades, there has been an enormous amount of research into the aetiology of ADHD. What we have found is that ADHD does sometimes run in families; there is a genetic component. There is good evidence demonstrated in twin studies that show a heritable component of the condition, but that does not tell the whole story. The genetic risks implicated in ADHD tend to have small effect sizes and cannot be used for genetic testing or diagnostic purposes beyond what is predicted by family history (Thapar, Cooper, Eyre, & Langley, 2013).

There is some evidence of structural (shape and size) and functional (activity) brain differences in people diagnosed with ADHD. The condition has been described as affecting the 'frontal' circuitry of the brain due to associated deficits in executive cognitive functioning: the thinking and processing regions of the brain (Wilens & Spencer, 2010). Brain imaging studies have identified differences in the size and shape of specific parts of the brain and the thickness of the folds of brain matter in children and adults with ADHD compared to those without the condition (Castellanos et al., 2002). Therefore, ADHD is thought to be mainly due to differences in the fine-tuning of the normal brain.

Just as some people may inherit a susceptibility to develop the symptoms of ADHD from their biological parents, there may be other likely causes. These may be infections, viruses or the effects of air pollution that cause problems with brain development while in the womb. The possibility also exists that there are undiscovered biological causes that influence the typical development of the central nervous system. Likewise, some authors suggest that psychosocial factors play a role in the expression of ADHD as we know it today. No single risk factor explains the condition with sufficient reliability yet, and opinions are often divided on the precise causes. ADHD, just like autism, is likely to have multiple origins and complex interactions with other conditions.

Diagnosis of ADHD

For a person to be diagnosed with ADHD, their symptoms should be associated with at least a moderate degree of psychological, social and educational or occupational impairment (NICE, 2018). Diagnosis is usually made by a specialist practitioner, psychiatrist, paediatrician or other healthcare professional and should be based on a full clinical and psychosocial assessment. The practitioner conducting the evaluation that informs the diagnosis will discuss the child's behaviour and symptoms across different settings of the child's everyday life. They will usually review a full developmental and psychiatric history, observer reports and an assessment of mental state.

The process of diagnosis is typically informed by a multi-agency team including Educational Psychologists, teachers, SENCOs and other professionals. Parents should be involved in this process and informed of the assessment progress and diagnostic outcomes and implications.

Diagnosis is made when symptoms of hyperactivity-impulsivity and inattention meet the criteria in either the DSM or ICD diagnostic manuals. There are specific diagnostic criteria for ADHD in the DSM and Hyperkinetic Disorder in the ICD diagnostic manuals. However, the reality is different from merely identifying a certain number of symptoms present before a given time and across settings.

As the cut-off between normal but difficult temperament and ADHD is not precisely definable, and there is no single reliable test for ADHD, the clinician's judgement plays a vital role in the diagnostic process. The clinician's experience and skill are critical to the diagnostic process, supported by evidence gathering in the form of assessments and clinical case history. The diagnostic process is typically based on taking information, observing symptoms, talking to the parents or carers, and seeing the child interacting with others in a variety of settings.

The Developmental Course and Lifespan of ADHD

ADHD persists across the lifespan, with most children first diagnosed around primary school age in the UK, that is from around the age of seven years old. ADHD can be characterised as a developmental disability; this suggests that it impairs the typical path of development. Therefore, we would expect typically-developing children to do just that, to 'typically develop'. However, in children diagnosed with ADHD, there is a change to that developmental pathway, usually expressed as some form of educational or behavioural consequence. Typically, these children are hindered in their school progression in some way or are singled out because of their behaviour. This expression of markers for ADHD is different for each child, and just as individual as factors such as the child's personality or disposition are.

Living with and caring for a child diagnosed with ADHD can be extremely difficult. There is likely to be additional stress on the family and challenges throughout the child's education if their condition is untreated. Having ADHD has severe consequences both in childhood and for some later into adult life. Follow-up studies of people diagnosed with ADHD suggest that they are far more likely than those without a diagnosis to repeat school years or drop out of school (Fried et al., 2016). People with ADHD are also more likely to get lower grades (Gormley, DuPaul, Weyandt, & Anastopoulos, 2016) and have friendships of shorter duration (Marton, Wiener, Rogers, & Moore, 2015) than people without a diagnosis. Later in life, they are also far more likely than others to underperform at work, to engage in anti-social activities, to use tobacco or illicit drugs, to have multiple car accidents, and to experience depression or personality disorders (Barkley et al, 2002).

Children with ADHD are not naughty because of their character; they are children with a disability. The challenges they face can range from mild to moderate learning and behavioural difficulties to very severe difficulties that stop them interacting with peers and learning at school. How the symptoms of ADHD affect each child is individually determined; the developmental course of ADHD is unpredictable, and each child is affected to a varying degree of severity. However, some markers of the condition, such as anxiety, are more commonly reported than others throughout the lifespan.

Preschool and Nursery

During the preschool and nursery years, children who are subsequently diagnosed with ADHD report a very short attention span; for example, not being able to listen for a long time. Likewise, moodiness and fine motor skill problems are reported, along with not being interested in playing with other children and poor self-control when frustrated or angry.

Infancy

Later in infancy and the toddler years, these children can be highly irritable and cry more frequently than other children. They can have sleep problems associated with being overactive and restless in the day. They may have difficulty adapting well to changes in the environment, be fussy eaters or have had difficulty nursing and feeding. Temperamental differences are sometimes noticed in infants where there is more than one young child in the family and comparisons are naturally made between them.

Primary School Years

The condition is typically diagnosed in the primary school years. It is here that children may fall behind in academic performance and may have trouble following rules and sitting quietly. Likewise, they may find it hard to pay attention and may have difficulty working cooperatively or productively with others for the first time.

Secondary School Years

At secondary school, these children may be characterised by their academic difficulties, especially with literacy. They may challenge parents' or teachers' authority and may have poor self-management or time-awareness, leading them to be frequently late or to fail to complete homework. They can be forgetful and easily bored; they may seem impulsive and irritable, and their apparent immaturity can lead them to high-risk behaviours. Many strategies and adaptations to make school life easier to engage with can be made to the child's environment.

Adults with ADHD

ADHD should be considered in all age groups: it is a lifelong condition. Of the young people with severe symptoms and a sustained diagnosis, many will go on to have significant difficulties in adulthood, which may include continuing ADHD, personality disorders, emotional and social difficulties, substance misuse, unemployment and involvement in crime. Likewise, many people later in life who are being treated for other health problems or who present directly to their local General Practitioners have been found to have undiagnosed ADHD.

For adults, who present with moderate or severe symptoms but who do not have a childhood diagnosis and where other psychiatric diagnoses do not explain these symptoms, it is typical to be referred to an ADHD specialist assessment centre. Clinicians will adjust symptom criteria for age-appropriate changes in behaviour at the point of evaluation, and details of the person's life history and early childhood will be examined for indications of ADHD. Similarly, coexisting conditions, social, familial, educational and occupational circumstances and physical health will be considered.

Of those people who do receive a diagnosis in childhood, some carry at least some symptoms into adulthood, although these may not always be problematic. These difficulties may manifest in adulthood as, for example, trouble with directions, having poor sustained attention, or finding it difficult to shift smoothly between activities. In adulthood, people with ADHD may frequently find themselves becoming distracted, may often lose things or may gain a reputation for continually fidgeting and interrupting other people. The transition from childhood ADHD to adulthood may be one of adaptation to and accommodation of the symptoms; some people find ways of coping, whereas some may have enduring problems into and throughout their adult life.

The estimated prevalence of adult ADHD is about 4-5 percent, although it has been found that the majority of adults with ADHD do not receive treatment directly for ADHD but are obtaining treatment for other co-morbid mental and substance-related disorders (Kessler et al., 2006). Surprisingly, one study showed that 90 percent of adults with ADHD lacked a history of any symptoms in childhood, suggesting that the condition may have to be reconsidered as a childhood-onset neurodevelopmental disorder (Moffitt et al., 2015).

Long-Term Outcomes for People with ADHD

When a child has ADHD, their symptoms can often be misunderstood as another condition or can exist alongside behavioural and conduct problems that may be due to reasons unrelated to inattention or hyperactivity. The primary markers of ADHD do not themselves cause behavioural issues; they are often confounded by the child's environment if it is poorly suited to their attentional needs and activity levels. In these children's formative years, they may get into trouble or be excluded from school; they may be bullied or may become bullies themselves.

With a vast range of possible troublesome consequences, it is crucial that children and adults with ADHD receive timely and appropriate diagnoses and support. With appropriate early identification, intervention, strategies and treatment, the prognosis is extremely good for most people who receive a diagnosis. Simple adaptations to the child's immediate environment at school and home can improve their ability to fulfil their potential in all areas of functioning.

As people diagnosed with ADHD pass into adulthood, leave the family home and gain employment, most manage and cope with their symptoms by adapting their occupations and home lives to suit. The long-term outcomes for people with childhood-onset ADHD are positive if the condition is addressed. However, many people with ADHD can have problems into adult life. In an extensive systematic review of 127 separate long-term studies, it was found that, compared to people without ADHD, most people with untreated ADHD had poorer self-esteem and social function. Treatment for ADHD, either medication or behavioural interventions was associated with an improvement in outcomes (Harpin, Mazzone, Raynaud, Kahle, & Hodgkins, 2016).

We will look at Autism Spectrum Disorder and Asperger's in more detail in Chapter 3.

Resources

For more information about ADHD and related conditions, visit the ADHD Foundation at their website:

www.adhdfoundation.org.uk.

The National Institute for Health and Care Excellence provides high-quality, evidence-based information to practitioners about ADHD on their website:

www.nice.org.uk/guidance/qs39.

If you would like to consider taking part in research studies about autism and ADHD, please visit www.ASDresearch.org to register your interest.

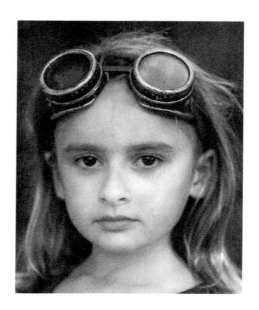

Chapter 3 – Autism Spectrum Disorder and Asperger's

When you have studied this chapter, you will understand and be able to describe the main symptoms, variations and diagnostic criteria for Autism and Asperger's Syndrome.

Key Points

- Autism is a lifelong developmental condition that is usually first diagnosed in childhood and affects people to varying degrees of severity in many ways across all areas of life.
- A person with autism typically has difficulty communicating and interacting with other people and may have characteristically repetitive patterns of behaviour and specialist or narrow areas of interests or activities.
- Asperger's Syndrome is a type of autism that is often less apparent in the social or communication areas of a person's life, although there may be social awkwardness, peculiarities in

27

spoken language and fixation with an obscure topic or specialist area of interest.

- Some people with autism may live very successful independent lives, and others will require a lifetime of specialist residential support.
- Individuals with all forms of autism across the spectrum of difficulties show the characteristics of the condition in different ways, and much can be done to alleviate the difficulties they face in society.

What is Autism?

There is a confusing excess of terms that cover a variety of presentations of the autism spectrum, such as, for example, Autistic Disorder, Asperger's Syndrome (or Disorder), High-Functioning, Pervasive Developmental Disorder (PDD), Semantic-Pragmatic Disorder, Pathological Demand Avoidance, Non-Verbal Learning Disability, Pervasive Developmental Disorder Not Otherwise Specified (PDD-NOS) and Atypical Asperger's Syndrome.

From early accounts, autism has been widely considered to exist across a continuum whereby it can be found with varying degrees of impairment and functioning, especially in *social interaction* (Wing & Gould, 1979). Now, autism is understood as a developmental condition that can significantly affect a person's verbal and non-verbal communication, social interactions, and education performance.

It is apparent before three years of age that children with autism are different from other, typically developing children. Characteristics include engagement in repetitive activities and so-called 'stereotyped' movements, resistance to environmental change or changes in daily routines, and unusual responses to sensory experiences. Autism affects a person's social interactions and communication and may lead to repetitive behaviours and obsessive interests.

Many people prefer the term *Autism Spectrum Condition* rather than *Autism Spectrum Disorder*, as it appears less stigmatising and it reflects that people with autism have not only disabilities that require a medical diagnosis but also areas of cognitive strength (Baron-Cohen et al., 2009).

The way autism is described in the public domain is different to the terms used to diagnose autism. It is important to note that the use of the term 'disorder' relates to a specific diagnostic property of the categorical 'medical model' approach of the Psychiatric diagnostic manuals used for classifying conditions. There is an increasing trend to use this phrase only to refer to the diagnostic category and to avoid using this phrase directly about individuals.

According to medical descriptions, autism is a syndrome; a cluster of symptoms appearing in a combination and a spectrum of markers that exist with varying severity. There is the presence of markedly atypical or delayed development in social interaction and communication and a markedly restricted repertoire of activities and interests. People with the condition typically have difficulties in areas that are well defined in the diagnostic manuals used for identifying the symptoms across the spectrum (American Psychiatric Association, 2000; World Health Organization, 1993). Other features that are often present include an insistence on sameness; attentional and perceptual abnormalities (e.g. people with autism can often notice fine details and tiny changes in their environments); and difficulties generalising learning to new situations.

To varying degrees, a person with autism is often overwhelmed with sensory information from their environment and may appear to retreat into their world or to engage in repetitive or controllable and familiar behaviours to cope. Some people with autism demonstrate so-called 'islets of ability', sometimes called 'savant abilities', who may be gifted at music, mathematics or drawing, for example. These talents and sometimes extreme abilities represent the minority of people across the autistic spectrum but seem to capture much public and media attention.

Many individuals with autism have a narrow band of interests that they may focus on obsessively; this may lead them to become extremely competent at a particular ability over time. For an even smaller proportion of people with these abilities, there may be brain-based explanations for their extreme expertise, and these individuals are of much interest to researchers but do not represent the overwhelming proportion of people with autism, who may show a narrow focus of interests and yet no savant abilities.

Characteristics of Autism

Sensory, emotional, social and attentional factors and self-awareness all play a part in the expression of the symptoms of autism. Many of the issues seen in autism are due to sensory overload from the environment causing the person with autism to withdraw into their world. The person with autism may prefer not to engage with social opportunities and may have poorer self-awareness.

The constant flood of sensations, a hypersensitivity to the world around them that overwhelms the person, can lead to 'meltdowns' or tantrums. Stimming, flapping and repetitive movements give the person with autism some control over their sensory processing and are predictable and are often prevalent when they are overcome with anxiety through sensory overload. The special interests of the person are the familiar things that they allow into their world, and these typically help them to feel safe and have relief from some of the anxiety that they may feel.

In young children, the markers of autism can vary, but there are a few commonly reported characteristics, such as reduced eye contact; not seeming to know how to play with toys; excessively lining up toys or other objects; attaching to one toy or object, and not smiling. At times, the child may seem to be hearing impaired and may fail to point at objects or to make baby babble or gestures by one year of age. Very early on, the child may not respond to their name when called or may develop and then lose some language or social skills. Likewise, there may be hypersensitivity (over) or hyposensitivity (under) to sounds, tastes, sights, smells or the tactile sensation of clothes, and the child may favour certain clothes or foods over others. Children with autism may prefer not to be held or cuddled or may cuddle only when they want to. Some people with autism have trouble relating to others and show little interest in other people at all.

As with ADHD, the person with autism may be prone to interpreting language overly literally. For example, in a story where a fictional Police Officer says 'Freeze!', the person with autism may be confused. This confusion may persist where figurative language, metaphor and literal language is used. Some individuals with autism report a qualitatively different way of thinking, for example sometimes reporting that they 'think in pictures'. This way of characterising autism as a difference rather than a disability is optimistic and allows the positive qualities of autism to be recognised and celebrated.

Conventionally autism has been characterised by difficulties across three primary areas that provide a broad yet imprecise way of thinking about what autism is:

i)   *Social Interaction.*
ii)   *Verbal and Non-verbal Communication.*
iii)   *Social Imagination – Restricted, Repetitive and Stereotyped Patterns of Behaviour.*

This so-called 'Triad of Impairment' (Wing & Gould, 1979) summarises the difficulties for the person with autism and historically has been a foundation for the diagnostic criteria set out in the DSM and ICD diagnostic manuals. However, the presentation of the classic symptoms of autism is dependent on the individual and the setting they find themselves in.

Difficulties in Social Interaction

Troubles comprehending the world around them can result in people with autism appearing to have behaviours that are peculiar or anti-social, and the person with autism may seem to withdraw entirely or may attempt to interact but may upset, bore or irritate others. People with autism may have profound difficulties in initiating and maintaining friendships and social relationships, and there can be an absence of spontaneous seeking to share enjoyment, interests or achievements with others. For parents, this relationship can be frustrating, particularly where there are other children in the household, with which comparisons naturally are made.

Difficulties in Verbal and Non-verbal Communication

Most people with autism also have problems with their receptive (understanding) and expressive (spoken and written) language. Some people with autism are non-verbal (about 15 percent), but this is not an indication that they cannot understand words spoken to them. Even if the person does have functional language proficiency, they can still have difficulty spontaneously producing, interpreting and responding to non-verbal cues and interpreting spoken language.

Most people on the autism spectrum have some difficulty interacting with others. They may appear not to hear what is said to them, fail to respond to their name or appear indifferent to any attempts to communicate with them. Young children especially may show echolalia (the repetition of other people's words), but this may also indicate that the child's communication is developing. Understanding the communicative expression of a person with autism can be essential to support them. The public and experts alike can learn as much from the autistic's world as they can from the 'neurotypical' world. Differences rather than disabilities, in communication, perception and thinking are often the most apparent.

The National Autistic Society has more information on communicating on their website: http://cms.autism.org.uk/about/communication.aspx.

Difficulties in Social Imagination – Restricted, Repetitive and Stereotyped Patterns of Behaviour

People with autism can find changes to routine or familiar circumstances challenging to cope with. Structure and organised systems and schedules assist the ability to make sense of the sensory overload reported by many people with autism. This ability to retreat to familiar interests or routines provides the safety and comfort of regular and predictable occurrences under the control of the individual. In younger children, hand 'flapping' or 'stimming' can allow them some predictable control over their environments when stressed by overwhelming stimuli around them. Likewise, people with autism often develop obsessive interests and rigid and restricted behavioural patterns and can become very set in their routines.

In this last category, of restricted, repetitive patterns of behaviour, we see some of the markers that are more specific to autism. These are behaviours such as the stereotyped hand and finger gestures, peculiar voice intonation, and preoccupation with objects that can characterise their obsessions or special interests. In children, these intense interests can be specialist subjects like, for example, 'Thomas the Tank Engine', dinosaurs or historical events. Likewise, they may use unusual body posturing or repeat actions or movements repeatedly or have compulsive behaviours such as lining up toys or twisting and spinning objects, which they may find highly stimulating or curious. There may also be a strong desire for sameness and anxiety when routines such as the daily schedule or familiar, immediate surroundings are changed.

The move towards an improved understanding and appreciation of the full range of symptoms and the uniqueness of the person with autism is helping with greater acceptance of the condition in society. The *Triad of Impairment* helps to summarise the difficulties for the autistic child, but the actual manifestation of these can vary considerably.

New Diagnostic Criteria for Autism Spectrum Disorder

Although early descriptions of autism, such as the *Triad*, can be helpful in describing some of the issues of people with autism, we have moved towards a much better understanding of the condition in recent years.

The significant change to the diagnosis of Asperger's Disorder and Autistic Disorder in the most recent version of the diagnostic manual is the use of the umbrella term 'Autism Spectrum Disorder' within the DSM-5 (American Psychiatric Association, 2013). The term 'Asperger's Syndrome' or 'Asperger's Disorder' as it appeared in the DSM-IV is no longer used for new diagnoses under these criteria, although people with an existing diagnosis retain this. The age of onset is more flexible, allowing for older children and adults to be diagnosed.

In the latest version of the diagnostic manual, the key features that represent the group of markers presented in autism were revised to include just two primary areas, forming a 'Dyad' (American Psychiatric Association, 2013):

i) Social Communication and Interaction.
ii) Restricted, Repetitive Patterns of Behaviour, Interests or Activities.

Social Communication and Interaction

The DSM-5 (American Psychiatric Association, 2013) refers to:

"Persistent deficits in social communication and social interaction across multiple contexts, as manifested by markers such as: Deficits in social-emotional reciprocity, ranging, for example, from abnormal social approach and failure of normal back-and-forth conversation; to reduced sharing of interests, emotions, or affect; to failure to initiate or respond to social interactions. Deficits in nonverbal communicative behaviours used for social interaction, ranging, for example, from poorly integrated verbal and nonverbal communication; to abnormalities in eye contact and body language or deficits in understanding and use of gestures; to a total lack of facial expressions and nonverbal communication. Deficits in developing, maintaining, and understanding relationships, ranging, for example, from difficulties adjusting behaviour to suit various social contexts; to difficulties in sharing imaginative play or in making friends; to absence of interest in peers."

Restricted, Repetitive Patterns of Behaviour, Interests or Activities

Likewise, the DSM-5 refers to:

"...restricted, repetitive patterns of behaviour, interests, or activities, as manifested by markers such as stereotyped or repetitive motor movements, use of objects, or speech (e.g., simple motor stereotypies, lining up toys or flipping objects, echolalia and idiosyncratic phrases). Insistence on sameness, inflexible adherence to routines, or ritualised patterns or verbal or nonverbal behaviour (e.g., extreme distress at small changes, difficulties with transitions, rigid thinking patterns, greeting rituals, need to take the same route or eat food every day). Highly restricted, fixated interests that are abnormal in intensity or focus (e.g., strong attachment to or preoccupation with unusual objects, excessively circumscribed or perseverative interest). Hyper- or hypo-reactivity to sensory input or unusual interests in sensory aspects of the environment (e.g., apparent indifference to pain/temperature, adverse response to specific sounds or textures, excessive smelling or touching of objects, visual fascination with lights or movement)."

These new 'domains' of autism under the DSM-5 criteria are each specified with three levels of severity or 'dimensional elements' to the diagnosis of autism, which indicate how much someone's condition affects them across social communication impairments and restricted, repetitive patterns of behaviour.

The Dimensional Elements (levels of severity) for autism are:

Level 1 – 'Requiring Support'.

Level 2 – 'Requiring Substantial Support'.

Level 3 – 'Requiring Very Substantial Support'.

In the ICD-10 diagnostic manual, autism is categorised by the presence of social and communication difficulties, alongside unusually strong, narrow interests and/or repetitive and stereotyped behaviour (World Health Organization, 1993). The next version of the ICD will largely duplicate the latest DSM-5 diagnostic criteria for Autism Spectrum Disorder.

What is Asperger's Syndrome?

For the person with Asperger's Syndrome, the profile is typically somewhat different, with the main challenges they face being with social interaction alongside subtle peculiarities with verbal and non-verbal communication, rather than significant language impairment.

Asperger's Syndrome, also known as 'Asperger's Disorder' or 'Asperger Syndrome', is a type of autism where cognitive ability (intelligence) is usually in the average or superior range, and there is no language delay (e.g., single words by two years; phrase speech by three years). Autism is a spectrum of conditions across a broad range of abilities and weaknesses, with Asperger's Syndrome often described as being towards the 'higher-functioning' end; although the use of that term is contentious and fails to acknowledge that the condition can have a profound impact on a person's life and relationships.

Asperger's Syndrome is mostly a hidden disability in the sense that people typically cannot tell that someone has the condition from his or her outward appearance. The condition is characterised by difficulties interacting socially with others and by some peculiarities in speech and language comprehension, but no significant learning difficulties. A person with Asperger's may have inflexible or rigid behaviours and intense interests, which can lead to lots of knowledge about a specialist topic. Individuals with Asperger's Syndrome tend to desire to interact with others but can have difficulties knowing how to do so in an appropriate way.

Some see Asperger's Syndrome as a more subtle form of the condition than so-called 'classic' presentations. Although it is frequently suggested that Asperger's comprises an entirely different condition, there continue to be mixed feelings in the community and among professionals about the formal inclusion of 'Asperger's Disorder' in the category 'Autism

Spectrum Disorder' within the DSM-5 diagnostic manual. Although in the DSM-5 the category title for autism is Autism Spectrum Disorder (ASD), many people prefer to use the term 'Autism Spectrum Condition' (ASC) or just 'autism', to reduce the emphasis on any negative elements.

People with Asperger's Syndrome frequently have difficulties with social interaction. This difficulty is often displayed as problems in the use of multiple nonverbal behaviours, such as eye-to-eye gaze, facial expression, body postures and gestures to regulate social interaction; failure to develop peer relationships appropriate to developmental level; and a lack of social or emotional reciprocity. The condition is also characterised by restricted, repetitive and stereotyped patterns of behaviour, interests and activities, as demonstrated by such things as a preoccupation with one or more stereotyped and restricted patterns of interest that are abnormal either in intensity or focus; there may be an apparently inflexible adherence to specific, non-functional routines or rituals and stereotyped and repetitive motor mannerisms.

Asperger's Syndrome is a lifelong disorder of unknown origin that usually shows up around 18 months to three years of age. It is thought to be a form of autism and is characterised by normal or above-normal intelligence; social awkwardness; verbal rigidity; and fixation with an obscure topic that can be learned by rote. People with Asperger's Syndrome have a hard time relating to other people. They may talk for hours about their obsessions or special interests. As children, they may not be interested in playing with other children. They can have a preoccupation with things that seem beyond their age level and show little or no eye contact.

A person with Asperger's Syndrome may talk with flat affect (they may sound 'robotic'), and their voice and tone modulation may fail to make their voice interesting to the listener because they lack the concept of the listener as interested. Their speech may be characterised by poor prosody, awkward intonation and odd/inappropriate subject matter.

People with Asperger's are inclined to construe language very literally, so they may not understand slang, informal speech or may find jokes that depend on dual-meanings hard to understand or fail to see the humour in them. They may also have difficulty decoding and understanding people's tone of voice and facial expressions especially where these rely on sarcasm or wittiness.

Unlike people with 'classic' profiles of autism, who may sometimes seem aloof and disinterested in others, people with Asperger's tend to desire to interact with others but lack the skills to do so in an appropriate way. People with Asperger's are often self-described 'loners' but may live very successful independent lives in appropriate job settings or may choose to live alone or prefer the company of pet animals. The very characteristics that make an individual 'higher functioning' can produce unique difficulties for a person with Asperger's Syndrome in all areas of their life. For example, because the markers are less visible, their difficulties may not always be taken seriously by others; likewise, there may be a much later diagnosis, or at school, they may not always be disruptive, although they may seem extremely intelligent. The condition is easy to miss or misdiagnose, and teachers may misunderstand the condition for misbehaviour more generally.

Prevalence of Autism

In her classic work *'Autism: Explaining the Enigma'*, Uta Frith states:

> "Autism is not a modern problem, even though it has only been recognised in modern times. In view of the short history of psychiatry, and the even shorter history of child psychiatry, we know that a disorder recently described is not necessarily a recent disorder. An increase in diagnosed cases does not necessarily mean an increase in cases."

(Frith, 2003, p. 34).

The reports of prevalence vary wildly, but autism is now thought to be more common than childhood Cancer, Down's Syndrome, Spina Bifida or Cystic Fibrosis. Around one out of every 68 families will have a child on the autism spectrum. Studies show that approximately 1 percent of UK children are on the autism spectrum, including Asperger's Syndrome (Baron-Cohen et al., 2009). This is a 12-fold increase in estimates from 1978 (Rutter, 1978).

A strikingly higher prevalence of autism than previous estimates was found in a survey of all of South Korea's 7–12-year-old children (Kim et al., 2011). This study showed that approximately one child in every 38, nearly 3 percent, in mid-childhood has some degree of autism. Worryingly, two-thirds of the children in this study who were identified as being on the autism spectrum who were in mainstream schools were undiagnosed and received no specific support for autism. The researchers argue that these findings suggest that rigorous large-scale screening is needed to produce more-accurate autism prevalence estimates and to underscore the need for better detection, assessment and services.

It is unclear how much of the increase in cases of autism is due to a broader definition, awareness and better efforts in diagnoses. However, an actual increase in the number of people with autism cannot be ruled out. The increase in autism diagnoses is likely due to a combination of these factors.

Gender Differences in Autism

Autism is more common in males; Boys are reportedly referred for help about four times as often as Girls, but it is not entirely known as to why. Although, this may be due to some of the same reasons why boys are more likely to be diagnosed with ADHD; their behaviour is typically more disruptive than that of girls. Girls may be more withdrawn and internalise their reactions and typically have more extensive social groups, possibly masking any issues with social interactions.

Girls on the autism spectrum present differently from boys, and research has long recognised that when girls have autism, they are likely to be more severely affected (Lord, Schopler, & Revicki, 1982). Educationalists in the school system, practitioners and parents should be aware of the possibility of autism in both boys and girls. Girls may be formally identified at a later age than boys, and this may delay referral for early intervention (Giarelli et al., 2010). Some researchers have argued that because boys differ in the presentation of symptoms from girls, diagnostic questions should be altered to identify some females on the autism spectrum who may otherwise be missed (Gould & Ashton-Smith, 2011). In an extensive study of people diagnosed with autism and Asperger's Syndrome, boys were much more likely to have hyperactivity or a short attention span and aggressive behaviour (Giarelli et al., 2010).

Other researchers suggest fundamental differences between the genders that relate strongly to the strengths and difficulties seen in some people with autism. In his classic book, *The Essential Difference* (2003), Simon Baron-Cohen argues that 'female-type brains' are better at empathising, while 'male-type brains' are stronger at understanding and building systems of all kinds. He suggests that autism is a form of the extreme male psychological profile that may be related to higher than normal levels of prenatal testosterone. People with an *extreme male brain*, mostly men, tune into tiny details or facts and are less concerned with social chit-chat or other people's points of view; they have less empathy and higher 'systemising'. At its extremes, Baron-Cohen suggests this profile is what we know as autism.

Differences Across the Spectrum

Asperger's Syndrome typically has a later onset and a higher range of intelligence quotient (IQ). There is no significant language deficit, and the difficulties in non-verbal communication problems are less severe than in other forms of autism. There may be clumsiness in basic motor skills. This profile contrasts subtly with the traditional presentation of autism, which is sometimes referred to as 'classic autism'.

The classic depiction of autism, which historically was the first to be identified, is characterised by a spectrum of ability and disability that can vary in its presentation and severity of impairment. Difficulties are present across all people with autism but being autistic will affect the individual in different ways. Autistics can be represented on this spectrum by their wide variety of capabilities both within themselves and in relation to others. All forms of autism affect a person's social interaction, communication, interests and behaviour in different ways and it is best to characterise autism as a *difference* rather than a disorder in this respect.

Some individuals with autism fail to develop spoken language, and there are always difficulties with verbal and non-verbal communication. The main difference between Asperger's Syndrome and 'Classic' autism is mainly in language development: typically, people with Asperger's Syndrome will not have had delayed language development when younger.

Conditions that often occur with Autism

Autism rarely occurs in isolation from other conditions. In addition to the primary diagnostic indicators of autism, many people will also exhibit a variety of other conditions and symptoms alongside autism. These are conditions such as tics (blinking, sniffing, facial grimaces and throat clearing); sensory sensitivities; Obsessive-Compulsive Disorder; executive dysfunction; ADHD; anxiety; sleep disturbances; eccentric or restrictive eating habits; self-injurious behaviours; Depression, especially in adolescents; and sometimes learning disabilities (intellectual disability), even though they may not be formally diagnosed with these conditions.

The Causes and Risk Factors for Autism

Many research centres around the world are looking at the causes of autism. However, scientific investigation has some way to go before we can specify the exact causes of autism. In line with the notion that there may be many different types of autism is the recognition that there may be many different causes of autism. Children who have a brother or sister diagnosed with autism are at a much higher risk of also having autism, and it has been established that genes are one of the risk factors that can make a person more likely to develop autism. There may be many different factors that make a child more likely to have autism, including their environment and biological and genetic (heritable) factors.

There are many plausible theories about the causes of autism that exist across different fields of enquiry, including biological and cognitive explanations. Underpinning these ways of understanding the causes of autism are many neurobiological studies in which specific brain areas are implicated in the markers of autism. In people with autism, problems in language and social development signpost the involvement of the limbic system, whereas motor problems suggest the involvement of the brainstem, cerebellum, thalamus and basal ganglia regions of the brain.

The 'Centers for Disease Control and Prevention' in the United States are conducting one of the most extensive research studies looking at many possible risk factors for autism, including genetic, environmental, pregnancy and behavioural factors.

You can find out more about this research here: www.cdc.gov/ncbddd/autism/research.html.

Diagnosis of Autism Spectrum Disorder

There are no definitive neurobiological markers for autism; there are no medical tests, such as blood tests or scanning tests that can be used for diagnosing the condition. Hence, it is primarily diagnosed by observed behaviour and clinical case history.

The time it takes for children to receive a diagnosis of autism in the UK varies across geographical regions (Local Authorities), but, currently, this can be as long as three and a half years. Guidelines from NICE recommend a maximum of three months between a referral and the first appointment for an autism assessment, but in some regions this routinely takes closer to 12 months. The wait for a diagnosis can be a stressful period for families, and this is a critical time for parents to understand the differences between autism and other conditions, and to prepare themselves with knowledge of the autism spectrum.

There are further information and support available on the NAS webpages: www.autism.org.uk.

Assessment

Assessment for diagnosis typically occurs in clinics, assessment centres, or private practices and is led by psychiatrists, psychologists or physicians. Assessment for suspected autism involves a thorough interview and gathering history from the patient and family, especially the patient's early development, to clarify the presence of critical areas of deficit and to rule out other conditions. A multidisciplinary team approach is best to evaluate language/pragmatics, cognitive, adaptive behaviour, social and familial, medical/neurological status, and sensory/motor issues.

Thorough assessment depends on information gathered through a variety of methods from professionals, family members and educators. Although there are many assessment tools to assist with diagnoses, there is not a single test that when used alone can provide a definitive diagnosis of autism.

Support for Autism

Ensuring people with autism get the best treatment and care is vital to positive long-term outcomes. While autism has no 'cure', early access to specialist treatment can help greatly. A diagnosis should not stand in the way of receiving treatment. The school Special Educational Needs and Disability process and the school's Co-ordinator (SENCo), along with the Local Authority (County Council), should provide adequate support for a child's individual needs.

For organisations, the NICE quality standard on autism highlights how organisations can ensure they are delivering the best treatment and support for people with this condition (National Institute for Health and Care Excellence, 2014).

National Autistic Society – 'Too Much Information' Campaign

The leading organisation for supporting people with autism and their carers, the National Autistic Society (NAS), recently ran the 'Too Much Information' campaign to focus on public understanding the condition. They emphasise that when being around someone on the autism spectrum, it is essential to give them time, as it can take a while to recover from information overload. They also recommend making space: trying to create a quiet, safe space as best you can. Other recommendations include asking people not to stare, to turn off loud music, and to turn down bright lights. It also helps to imagine feeling so overloaded that you could not cope.

If you suspect you or your child has autism or a related condition, you should consider making an appointment to see your local General Practitioner (GP) to discuss a referral to a Paediatrician or specialist assessment clinic.

We will look at classification, assessment and diagnosis in more detail in Chapter 4.

Resources

For more information about autism, visit the National Autistic Society at their website:

www.autism.org.uk.

For more information about autism research, therapies and interventions, visit Autistica at their website:

www.autistica.org.uk.

More information about the signs and symptoms of autism can be found on the Centres for Disease Control and Prevention website: http://www.cdc.gov/ncbddd/autism/facts.html.

The National Institute for Health and Care Excellence provides high-quality, evidence-based information to practitioners about autism on their website:

www.nice.org.uk/guidance/qs51.

If you would like to consider taking part in research studies about autism and ADHD, please visit www.ASDresearch.org to register your interest.

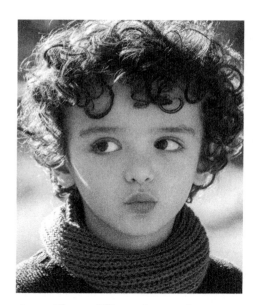

Chapter 4 – Classification, Assessment and Diagnosis

When you have studied this chapter, you will understand and be able to describe the central debates and ethical considerations of classification, assessment and diagnosis.

Key Points

- Autism and ADHD are diagnosed mainly on a behavioural and clinical case history basis.
- There is significant variation in symptoms, and the severity of impairments across individuals with these conditions differs greatly.
- Two diagnostic manuals (DSM, ICD) inform decision-making.
- There are multiple referral routes and multiple assessment tools.
- The process of being diagnosed can be long and can delay a person receiving appropriate support.

The Purpose of Classification

The 'Medical Model'

The 'medical model' treats mental conditions in the same way as fractured limbs and as such is somewhat guilty of suggesting an underlying physical (or neurological) disorder where none may exist. For autism and ADHD, we must be particularly cautious of such models and guarded when using the terminology employed in the diagnostic manuals that are essential to this way of grouping together clusters of commonly occurring characteristics into clinical categories. Both the ICD and DSM diagnostic manuals use a tick-list therapeutic approach. We do not conclusively know what causes autism or ADHD, so it may be fair to say that we cannot rely on clinical classification and diagnosis to be accurate all the time. Both Psychiatrists and Psychologists adopt this model when they refer to disorders as diseases and specific behaviour as symptoms.

However, categorising clusters of characteristics or markers (symptoms) into clinical diagnostic categories does give practitioners useful information about the prognosis of a condition and allows us to build up knowledge of successful treatments, strategies and adjustments for the condition. In short, the medical model makes it possible to relate tried-and-tested solutions with a reasonable degree of consistency. Thus, assessment leads us to diagnosis, which in turn leads to treatments that may relieve symptoms, even if we are unsure of the underlying causes of a condition.

It may be sufficient to say that people are different from one another, rather than suggest that a person has a 'disorder' because they deviate from the norm. For example, the so-called 'neurodiversity' movement challenges these assumptions about causation and cure and celebrates conditions such as these as an inseparable aspect of identity (Kapp, Gillespie-Lynch, Sherman, & Hutman, 2013). Many people, both on and off 'the spectrum' of autism, oppose research into the causes of autism and view autism as a different cognitive style – a different way of thinking. Therefore, we must be sensitive that there are differing opinions and perspectives on the benefits of a diagnosis, the need for assessment, and the ethics of 'treatment'.

The Purpose of Assessment

Assessment means measuring and observing a person's strengths and weaknesses to inform care plans and assist in reaching decisions about diagnosis, if appropriate. Assessments compare an individual's presenting behaviour, characteristics and abilities to developmental milestones that are typical of people of the same age. With adults, their current age is less a factor, and issues such as comparisons with social norms of behaviour are more informative, together with a record of their development and behaviour throughout childhood and later life. Assessment also informs the development of interventions and measures their effectiveness.

Specialist practitioners, doing assessments for diagnostic purposes, use their professional judgement and understanding of people with similar markers and characteristics alongside information such as a clinical case history, to reach an informed and evidence-based decision on the way forward. They will evaluate if a person's presenting 'symptoms' and clinical case history meet the required criteria set out in the diagnostic manuals and whether it is to the advantage of a person to receive a formal diagnosis. Assessment for these purposes is not about labelling the person; instead, it should be about information gathering and bringing together the available information to reach well-informed decisions about a possible diagnosis. In this way, assessments inform care strategies and treatment, as well as support the diagnostic process.

Assessing Autism

As well as a different way of thinking and seeing the world, autism can be thought of as a group of developmental disabilities that can cause significant social, communication and behavioural challenges, rather than as a single condition that presents the same characteristics in those with the condition. In this sense, autism can be extremely challenging to identify accurately, and there is no practical way to specify subtypes as there is with ADHD. Therefore, there is a tendency to specify the type of autism mainly by the levels of severity of impairment within the person.

Assessment of autism is likely to involve a specialist autism team talking with the parent and observing the child. They will seek to find out about i) the parent's concerns, ii) how the child has been getting on at home, nursery or school, or in care, iii) the child's past and present health, and iv) the child's behaviour and development.

The National Institute for Health and Care Excellence (NICE) guidelines (2011) provide recommendations for the elements that should be established in the assessment process for autism for children and young people:

- Detailed questions about the parent's or carer's concerns and, if appropriate, the child's or young person's concerns.
- Details of the child's or young person's experiences of home life, education and social care.
- A developmental history, focusing on developmental and behavioural features consistent with ICD-10 or DSM-5 (current diagnostic manuals) criteria (consider using an autism-specific tool to gather this information).
- Assessment (through interaction with, and observation of the child or young person) of social and communication skills and behaviours, focusing on features consistent with ICD-10 or DSM-5 criteria (consider using an autism-specific tool to gather this information).
- A medical history, including prenatal, perinatal and family history, and past and current health conditions.
- A physical examination.

NICE guidelines for autism in adults have also been produced (2012).

Assessment is often compiled across a multidisciplinary team across several appointments with different specialists, who may gather information in a variety of ways. These may include reports from several settings (e.g. school, nursery and home), multi-site observations, specialist assessment tools, a full clinical case history, a physical examination, and tests and evaluations for other conditions, where appropriate. Following the process of evaluation, a report will be produced that will detail the specific diagnosis; test scores may be appended, and the report will usually indicate the course of action to be taken or recommendations. This report may come in a variety of forms, for example, a letter from a paediatrician, a specialist assessment centre or a specialist practitioner.

NICE provides a guide to recognition, referral and diagnosis: *CG128 Autism: Autism in under 19s* (2011), which informs the diagnostic process. Thorough assessment depends on information gathered through a variety of methods from specialist diagnosticians, the child's family and often teachers. A single source of information alone is not sufficient to provide adequate information from which to make a diagnosis.

Diagnosis should be conducted by a team of suitably trained professionals following quality standards for assessment and diagnosis; in turn, they will produce a personalised plan for the person with autism that coordinates care and support, which can involve treatment with psychosocial interventions and/or medication (NICE, 2014).

Assessment Tools for Autism

Diagnostic assessment tools for autism are used in the context of clinics, private practices or home visits and are conducted and interpreted by

Psychiatrists, Psychologists or physicians. A multi-method assessment approach is best, not just relying on one source of information (such as an observation) alone. Many different evaluation tools can be used to inform the data-gathering phase of an autism assessment and diagnosis.

Diagnosticians vary in the evaluation and diagnostic tools they are trained to use and favour. A clinician involved in diagnoses may use some or none of these, depending on the applicability of the measure and local practice. Some practitioners rely more heavily on interviewing the parents and carers, and some use other methods such as observation or interactions with the child, which are interpreted or analysed considering behaviours and markers for the condition.

One frequently used assessment tool is the Autism Diagnostic Interview-Revised (ADI-R) (Lord, Rutter, & Le Couteur, 1994), which is a standardised, semi-structured parent interview that lasts about 1½ hours and is valid from 18 months into adulthood. A parent is asked to describe their child's past and current behaviour, focusing on preschool years. It is scored using an algorithm highly consistent with DSM and ICD criteria. It can help to inform the process of diagnosis, but, like all other assessment tools, it cannot be relied on in isolation.

Examples of other assessment tools for autism include:
- The Diagnostic Interview for Social and Communication Disorders (DISCO).
- The Childhood Autism Rating Scale (CARS).
- The Autism Screening Questionnaire (ASQ).
- The Checklist for Autism in Toddlers (CHAT).
- The Screening Test for Autism in Two-Year-Olds (STAT).
- The Adolescent Autism Spectrum Quotient (AQ).
- The Adult Asperger Assessment (AAA).
- The Autism Diagnostic Observation Schedule-Generic (ADOS-G).
- The Asperger Syndrome (and High-Functioning Autism)

Diagnostic Interview (ASDI).
- The Ritvo Autism Asperger Diagnostic Scale-Revised (RAADS-R).

Shorter screening assessments can also be used to determine whether further diagnostic testing for autism is warranted.

Early Indicators of Autism

The National Institute of Child Health and Human Development (NICHD) lists behaviours that signal that further evaluation may be justified:

- Does not babble or 'coo' by 12 months.
- Does not gesture (point, wave and grasp) by 12 months.
- Does not say single words by 16 months.
- Does not say two-word phrases on his or her own by 24 months.
- Has any loss of any language or social skill at any age.

Likewise, within a child's first year, the presence of indicators may suggest that further evaluation is needed:

- Lack of eye contact to initiate joint attention.
- Emotionally distant behaviour or dislike of affection.
- Lack of imitation or social reciprocity.
- Lack of functional use of non-verbal communication.
- Inappropriate use of toys.

These indicators may further warrant screening for autism if a sibling or another family member has an existing diagnosis of autism.

Assessing ADHD

To ensure that an accurate diagnosis of ADHD is conducted, it is crucial that a full assessment be carried out by a healthcare professional with specialised training and expertise in ADHD. Individual assessment for

ADHD mostly follows the same types of procedure as that for autism but usually involves a dedicated team of professionals to deliver appropriate assessment tools and observations coupled with clinical experience. Symptoms suggestive of ADHD are often identified in children and young people by their GPs or teachers in the first instance.

The diagnostic process is typically based on taking information via a full clinical and psychosocial assessment of the person, observing symptoms, talking to the parents or carers, a full developmental history, and seeing the child interacting with others in a variety of settings. There is no single test for ADHD that can be reliably used in isolation to make a diagnosis. Although the DSM sets out the clinical diagnostic criteria for ADHD, the pressing question for the clinician is where the cut-off lies between normal but difficult behaviour and childhood pathology. The decision is informed heavily by context, case history and is mostly a matter of clinical judgement.

Assessment Tools for ADHD

ADHD is typically diagnosed in the primary-school years. As with autism, assessment for diagnosis typically occurs in Clinics, private practices or home visits and is usually led by Child Psychiatrists, Paediatricians, Psychologists or physicians.

Many of the available assessment tools use checklists of symptoms that closely follow the DSM and ICD diagnostic criteria. Assessment tools such as the Conners' Comprehensive Behavior Rating Scales (Conners, Pitkanen, & Rzepa, 2011) use a series of questions across many separate elements to build up a picture of the person's unique strengths and difficulties and go further than simply evaluating the core elements of the condition. The Conners' Rating Scale-Revised (CRS-R) is also a commonly used assessment for ADHD. The scales assess behaviours, emotions, and academic and social problems in children and young adults from six years up to the age of 18 years. Assessments such as these often come in

Parent, Teacher and Self-Report versions. These question-based assessments are most frequently informed by clinical experience and psychiatric or paediatric opinion and should not be used in isolation.

Examples of other assessment tools for ADHD include:

- The Child Behaviour Checklist (CBCL).
- The Strengths and Difficulties Questionnaire (SDQ).
- Vanderbilt ADHD Diagnostic Rating Scale (VADRS).
- The ADD-H Comprehensive Teacher/Parent Rating Scale (ACTeRS).
- Swanson, Nolan, and Pelham-IV Rating Scale (SNAP-IV).
- NICHQ Vanderbilt Assessment Scale - Teacher/Parent.

The process of diagnostic assessment for ADHD has become more streamlined and accurate over recent years with the use of Quantitative Behaviour (QB) tests. These typically involve computerised cognitive function tests and are useful in establishing the reasons why certain behaviours occur and can inform the clinician's judgement when conducting a diagnostic assessment.

The Purpose of Diagnosis

Diagnosis is the process of assigning someone who is presenting symptoms to a classification based on agreed-upon diagnostic definitions and a set of criteria. For ADHD and autism, diagnosis must be made on a behavioural basis: there are no genetic markers or cognitive or perceptual markers unique to either. A diagnosis is usually made on evidence from a clinical interview where appropriate, careful observation of behaviour, medical records and assessment tests.

Getting a formal autism or ADHD diagnosis can open access to the right support, as well as explaining why certain things are so challenging. For most, a diagnosis is a positive event, and many children with ADHD or autism and their families benefit from having a diagnosis. Some families view a diagnosis with a sense of relief, and it can explain much about the individual. Other families, while well informed and knowledgeable about diagnostic criteria and psychiatric conditions, actively choose not to pursue a diagnostic pathway for their children.

For autism and ADHD, the earlier children are identified, the sooner they can get the external services and support they may need to help them to reach their full potential. However, little population-based data exist on the identification of autism and ADHD among preschool-aged children. In the case of autism, the available data indicate that the prevalence of autism at four years old is about 30 percent lower than at age eight years old (Christensen et al., 2016).

Autism and ADHD often frequently together and there is considerable overlap of symptoms. One way to think about the autistic spectrum is to think of autism and Asperger's Syndrome as *internalising* conditions, where children socially withdraw − the so-called *'autistic bubble'*. However, this contrasts with ADHD, which can be thought of this as an *externalising* condition. Individuals with classic 'Predominately Combined-type' ADHD rarely 'go inside' of themselves as one may well find with people on the autism spectrum; these children are typically very active and frequently *'in your face'*, occupying the time and attention of all of those around them. This is the case with the combined form of ADHD and the 'Predominately Hyperactive-Impulsive type' of ADHD. However, this is not the case with the 'Predominantly Inattentive' form of ADHD, which may more closely resemble the social isolation apparent in many autistics.

We can see from the preceding example that the conditions are very different from one another, but the presenting symptoms may resemble elements of each other, contributing to much complexity in assessment, diagnosis and treatment. When we talk about the symptoms, it is important to realise that these may occur in every one of us to varying degrees in our everyday lives. However, the subclinical features of these conditions, although observable in many of us, should not be confused with the indicators for diagnosable conditions. For a condition to be diagnosed one of the requirements is that it causes severe and persistent problems for the person across multiple settings and does not get better over time, at least not in the short-term.

There are multiple routes for getting a diagnosis, and this is often started through a child's school via specialists employed by the Local Authority who are involved with Special Educational Needs (SEN). However, a local General Practitioner (GP) can refer an individual to other health professionals who can start the process that leads to a diagnosis. Ultimately, a diagnosis is a statement by an acknowledged authority that after evaluation agrees upon using a medical category to describe symptoms of a specific type, in a particular combination. A diagnosis is an abbreviated way to describe a set of commonly-seen symptoms in a person.

The Diagnostic Manuals (DSM and ICD)

Two main diagnostic manuals inform the work of clinicians involved in diagnosing children with psychiatric conditions and illnesses. These are i) the *Diagnostic and Statistical Manual of Mental Disorders*, now in its fifth version (DSM-5, 2013) and published by the American Psychiatric Association, and ii) the *International Statistical Classification of Diseases and Related Health Problems*, in its 10th revision (ICD-10, 1992) and issued by the World Health Organization. Although the ICD is in continual revision, the next version has been significantly delayed and was due to be updated sometime in 2018.

There have been several editions of the DSM since the 1950s; the most recent edition, DSM-5, was released in 2013. Although used for diagnostic criteria, the ICD is used to monitor the incidence and prevalence of diseases and other health problems, providing a picture of the general health situation of countries and populations; by contrast, the DSM primarily lists mental health conditions and is mainly used by clinicians and researchers to diagnose and classify mental disorders. The terminology and descriptions of mental health conditions vary across versions of these manuals.

ADHD in the DSM-IV

In the previous version, the DSM-IV (APA, 2000), ADHD was listed alongside other disruptive behaviour disorders, such as Conduct Disorder and Oppositional Defiant Disorder. Under-controlled or externalising behaviour characterises these (i.e. 'acting out': socially disruptive conduct that is inappropriate given the age of the child and/or the setting of the behaviour). Behaviour is typically distressing and/or annoying to those in the child's social environment and is characterised by a persistent pattern of inattention and/or hyperactivity/impulsivity that is more frequent and severe than typically observed in those at comparable levels of development. In the DSM-IV, symptoms had to be present before age seven years in at least two settings.

The diagnostic manual also included 'Not Otherwise Specified' (NOS) categories that allowed for a diagnosis when the full number of diagnostic markers were not present. It is important to know about this previous version of the DSM, not just from a historical perspective but also because most existing diagnoses were made using these criteria and much research uses these labels.

Autism in the DSM-IV

In the DSM-IV (APA, 2000), autism was called 'Autistic Disorder' and 'Asperger's Disorder' and was categorised as a 'Pervasive Developmental Disorder'. These childhood disorders were characterised by impairment in verbal and non-verbal communication and social interaction, and abnormalities that occur in the developmental process itself; development is not delayed but is atypical. 'Autistic Disorder' was listed alongside Asperger's Disorder, Rett's Disorder and Childhood Disintegrative Disorder.

As with ADHD, the DSM-IV manual also included 'Not Otherwise Specified' categories that allowed for a diagnosis when the full number of diagnostic markers were not present. It was only the forms of Autistic Disorder and Asperger's Disorder that formed the autism spectrum, and most people referred to these as 'autism spectrum conditions'. In common usage many people prefer the term 'condition' and see this as preferential to the term 'disorder', which is synonymous with illness.

Because Asperger's varies considerably across individuals, making a diagnosis can be challenging; it is usually identified later than 'classic' or profound autism is, and sometimes difficulties may not be recognised and diagnosed until adulthood. The view that Asperger's Syndrome is autism without any additional learning disability or significant problems with language may be helpful from a diagnostic point of view but scarcely presents an accurate representation of the two conditions.

ADHD in the ICD-10

The ICD-10 medical classification system refers to ADHD as 'Hyperkinetic Disorder': a term widely used in Europe but infrequently used in the United States. The diagnostic criteria set out for Hyperkinetic Disorder in the ICD-10 are narrower than in the DSM and include people with more severe symptoms and impairment.

For a diagnosis of Hyperkinetic Disorder, the ICD-10 necessitates that 'data' is gathered for both inattention and hyperactivity in more than one situation (e.g. home, school and clinic) and that these should be diagnosed if they are disproportionate to the child's age and the context in which these are observed. The ICD-10 criteria for ADHD specify a combination of overactive, poorly modulated behaviour with marked inattention and a lack of persistent task involvement. The symptoms must exist before six years of age and be of long duration; there must be impairment present in two or more settings and no presence of anxiety, mood affective disorders or schizophrenia (World Health Organization, 1992). The ICD-10 states that children of preschool age should only be diagnosed when there are extreme levels of hyperactivity.

Autism in the ICD-10

In the latest version of the ICD, autism and Asperger's Syndrome are categorised as Pervasive Developmental Disorders. Autism is called 'Childhood Autism' and is defined by the presence of abnormal or impaired development that is apparent before the age of three years, alongside marked impairments in reciprocal social interaction and communication and with the presence of restricted, stereotyped, repetitive behaviour (World Health Organization, 1992).

Asperger's Syndrome is characterised as having similar challenges to the reciprocal social interaction issues present in autism, alongside a restricted, stereotyped, repetitive repertoire of interests and activities. However, the ICD-10 states that Asperger's Syndrome differs from autism mainly in the fact that there is no general delay in language or cognitive development.

ADHD in the DSM-5

The current DSM-5 diagnostic criteria are like those in the previous version. The fifth edition of the DSM was released in 2013 and replaces the earlier version. ADHD is now placed in the Neurodevelopmental Disorders chapter of the DSM-5. The same primary 18 symptoms for ADHD, divided into two symptom domains (inattention and hyperactivity/impulsivity), are used in the DSM-5 as were used in the

DSM-IV. These require there to be at least six symptoms of inattention and/or hyperactivity across at least two contexts (e.g. school and home) that are causing significant impairment to the person and are persistent across time. Several inattentive or hyperactive/impulsive symptoms must now be present before the age of 12 years, rather than before seven years old. In the DSM-5, the former 'primary subtypes' have been replaced with 'presentation specifiers' that map directly to them.

Based on the types of symptoms, three presentations of ADHD can occur (American Psychiatric Association, 2013):

- **Combined Presentation**: if enough symptoms of both inattention and hyperactivity/impulsivity criteria were present for the past six months.
- **Predominantly Inattentive Presentation**: if enough symptoms of inattention, but not hyperactivity/impulsivity, were present for the past six months.
- **Predominantly Hyperactive/Impulsive Presentation**: if enough symptoms of hyperactivity/impulsivity, but not inattention, were present for the past six months.

The presentation of ADHD may change over time, in line with changing symptoms. For an adult diagnosis to be made, the individual only needs to meet five symptoms, instead of the six required for younger people. Importantly, a comorbid diagnosis of Autism Spectrum Disorder is now also allowed in parallel with a diagnosis of ADHD.

More information can be found here: www.cdc.gov/ncbddd/adhd/diagnosis.html.

Autism in the DSM-5

In the latest version of the DSM (American Psychiatric Association, 2013), Autistic Disorder and Asperger's Disorder are now replaced with a single category: 'Autism Spectrum Disorder' (ASD). This change reflects a scientific consensus that the previously separate disorders in the DSM-IV are a single condition with different levels of symptom severity. ASD is characterised by:

1) **Deficits in social communication and social interaction.**
2) **Restricted, repetitive behaviours, interests and activities.**

Because both components are required for a diagnosis of ASD, 'Social Communication Disorder' is diagnosed if no restricted, repetitive behaviours are present.

Under the DSM-5, the term 'Asperger's Disorder' (Syndrome) is no longer used to specify a new diagnosis. However, all existing diagnoses using this label are retained unless re-diagnosis occurs. A comorbid diagnosis of ADHD is now allowed when symptoms of both conditions co-occur.

It is valuable to be aware of the DSM criteria, as these are the benchmark used not only in diagnosis but also in defining inclusion criteria to many research studies. Research suggests that estimates of the number of children with autism may be lower using the current DSM-5 criteria than using the previous DSM-IV criteria (Maenner et al., 2014).

Best Practice in Assessment and Diagnosis

As part of the Department of Health in the United Kingdom, NICE produces a range of high-quality, evidence-based practice guidelines that organisations can use to improve the quality of care. These set the quality standard for best practice throughout the National Health Service (NHS) and the private sector in the UK. Every parent, carer and person working in a setting that meets people diagnosed with both autism and ADHD are likely to find these guidelines useful. Each standard consists of a prioritised set of specific, concise and measurable statements. They draw on existing guidance, which provides an underpinning, comprehensive set of recommendations, and are designed to support the measurement of improvement. It is the ideal, if not the reality that Local Authorities (County Councils), the NHS and private practice draw from these guidelines to provide coordinated services.

NICE Guidelines for Autism

The NICE (2014) *Quality Standard QS51* for autism maps out standards for the care of people with autism. It lists the assessment and referral pathways and procedures that should be followed when people seek help and support, as well as guidance on treatment. The NICE guidelines *CG128* (2011) are the clinical guidelines on the recognition, referral and diagnosis of autism in under 19s. The NICE guidelines *CG170* (2013a) are the definitive clinical guidelines on the support and management of autism in under 19s. The guidelines *CG142* (NICE, 2012) provide definitive clinical guidelines on the diagnosis and management of autism in adults.

These documents can be found at https://pathways.nice.org.uk/pathways/autism-spectrum-disorder.

NICE Guidelines for ADHD

The NICE *Quality Standard QS39* (2013) for ADHD maps out standards for the care of people with ADHD. It lists the assessment and referral pathways and procedures that should be followed when people seek help and support as well as guidance on treatment. The guidelines *NG87* (NICE, 2018) are the definitive clinical guidelines on the diagnosis and management of ADHD.

These documents can be found at https://pathways.nice.org.uk/pathways/attention-deficit-hyperactivity-disorder.

Referral, Diagnosis and Beyond

To get a referral for a specialist assessment of either autism or ADHD, a person can make an appointment with their family doctor or health visitor, in the case of young children. However, in school-age children, a referral for an assessment is most often initiated by the school by the Special Educational Needs Co-ordinator (SENCO) with the help of outside agencies, such as the Educational Psychology Service of the Local Authority and other healthcare professionals.

A child has Special Educational Needs if he or she has learning difficulties or disabilities that make it harder for him or her to learn than most other children of about the same age. Involvement with agencies outside of the school may follow with a report called an 'Education, Health and Care Plan' (EHCP). This plan covers children from birth up to the age of 25 years, where needed. These were formally called a 'Statement' of Special Educational Needs. In some cases, a child may be referred for formal assessment, and this may result in a diagnosis of a condition such as ADHD or autism.

The average age of referral and diagnosis for girls is typically reported as higher compared to that for boys, which may be due to problems in identifying symptoms of autism between the genders. A retrospective study of children and adults diagnosed with autism found no difference in the duration of assessment for males and females (Rutherford et al., 2016). The findings of this study may suggest that delays in the diagnosis of females occur before referral for assessment and add support that there is a general delay in recognising autism in young girls.

The diagnosis itself should not be a barrier to accessing support, which is usually provided by the child's school in the first instance. After that, support is usually provided by a graduated response, if necessary requesting specialist help from the Local Authority from Educational Psychologists or other specialist teams, sometimes the Child and Adolescent Mental Health Services (CAMHS), including Psychiatrists, Psychologists, Social Workers and Occupational Therapists or, if appropriate, the Primary Healthcare Team (e.g. in the UK, NHS doctors and nurses).

Local regions have different support services available from the statutory, voluntary or school-based sector, such as a National Health Service (NHS) trust, Local Authority, school or charitable organisation. These agencies will usually first establish what the concerns are and what has been tried within the local school provision and will most often work with schools for positive outcomes.

Getting a referral, assessment, diagnosis and ultimately dedicated specialist support can be a very long journey. How much support a family ultimately gets may depend on several factors, such as location, social class, education and income. Getting help from Local Authority services or the specialist, CAMHS is different depending on what region a person lives. Waiting times for assessment or services can vary considerably across the UK. Some parents decide to pay for a private psychological assessment and report, which can reduce the waiting time to access services.

Considerations of Diagnosis and Assessment

The NICE Quality Standard QS51 (2014) for autism recommend that people with possible autism who are referred to an autism team for a diagnostic assessment receive an evaluation within three months of their referral. NICE states that it is important that the assessment is conducted as soon as possible so that appropriate health and social care interventions, advice and support can be offered.

Ensuring those who are affected by autism are given access to support as quickly as possible can help to improve outcomes. The reality is that people may have to wait for years to receive a diagnosis of either ADHD or autism following a referral; after diagnosis, they may also face a considerable delay in accessing services.

It is easier to identify autism at the 'low-functioning' end of the spectrum, where the symptoms are more obvious than at the 'higher-functioning' end. For example, the symptoms can include 'stimming', repetitive movements or challenges to the individual with the complexities of social communication. 'High-functioning' children with autism, including those with Asperger's Syndrome, do often adapt more successfully to the 'neurotypical' world around them. Thus, many of the significant markers of the condition may be masked by a person who has learnt to appear no different from most others around them.

'Autism', like 'ADHD', is an umbrella term that relates to a cluster of symptoms that appear together. The symptoms of people with autism can be very dissimilar.

Some estimates suggest that 8 percent of adults in England have ADHD (McManus, Meltzer, Brugha, Bebbington, & Jenkins, 2009), but many people may never formally identify it in themselves or seek treatment. Non-diagnosed ADHD in the community may account for many instances of self-medication in the form of 'recreational' drug use, such as tobacco, cannabis or alcohol. Although one study showed that more than one-third of adolescents and young adults endorsed using cigarettes and substances for self-medication (Wilens et al., 2007), further research is needed to establish the validity of such suggestions and the link to ADHD and autism. Individuals with symptoms of ADHD may be more likely to use these substances, but the relationship may be mediated by the presence of Conduct Disorder (Flory, Milich, Lynam, Leukefeld, & Clayton, 2003).

ADHD is usually identified in school but can be mistaken for bad behaviour or misdiagnosed as another condition, potentially delaying the time it may take for an accurate diagnosis. Diagnosis of ADHD and autism is usually first made in childhood, but the process for adults is very similar to that of children. Assessment typically entails a thorough interview and history of the child and family, especially early development, to clarify the presence of the condition and to rule out other clinical 'disorders'.

Asperger's Syndrome usually has a later onset of apparent symptoms than autism or ADHD, with a higher range of intelligence quotient; there is usually no language deficit, and non-verbal communication problems are typically less severe than in 'classic' or forms of profound autism. Difficulty identifying the symptoms of Asperger's Syndrome can lead to misdiagnosis or delayed diagnosis; the average age at diagnosis is several years later than for 'classic' forms of autism.

Approximately 13 percent of the children ever diagnosed with autism are estimated to have lost the diagnosis, and parents of 74 percent of them believed that it had changed due to new information according to one study (Blumberg et al., 2015). The most-efficient intervention programmes begin early and establish a management strategy at a young age that can minimise later behavioural problems. Misdiagnosis or late diagnosis can be distressing for individuals and their families.

In an extensive UK survey, parents of children with Asperger's Syndrome reported longer delays and higher frustration in obtaining a diagnosis than those with a child with autism ('classic' autism). In the autism group, the average age of diagnosis was five and a half years, but in the Asperger's group, it was eleven years (Howlin & Asgharian, 1999). Diagnosis can be missed or even misdiagnosed in individuals, and it may take many years to receive a diagnosis after first suspecting an individual has a condition such as ADHD or autism. There are multiple referral routes to assessment, and these may result in a person remaining on an evaluation waiting list for many months and sometimes years.

Thorough evaluation depends on information gathered through a variety of methods: from professionals, family members and a child's school teachers. There are multiple assessment tools, and although these may use clear criteria from the diagnostic manuals, the reality is different: this evaluation may rely mainly on a clinician's judgement, informed by additional evidence gathered from questionnaires, observations and clinical case history. Children's developmental trajectories are mostly unpredictable from diagnosis using the tick-list approach.

The cut-off between normal but difficult temperament and ADHD is not precisely definable, and assessment performance in a clinician's office or assessment centre is often weaker than it is either at school or at home in familiar settings. Factors such as these can make assessment and diagnosis of autism and ADHD challenging.

We will look at the theories and causes of autism and ADHD in more detail in Chapter 5.

Resources

For more information about the DSM diagnostic manual published by the American Psychiatric Association, see their website:

https://www.psychiatry.org.

For more information about the ICD diagnostic manual published by the World Health Organization, see their website:

http://apps.who.int/classifications/icd10.

If you would like to consider taking part in research studies about autism and ADHD, please visit www.ASDresearch.org to register your interest.

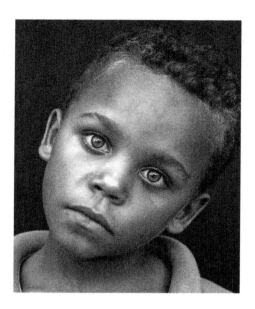

Chapter 5 – Theories and Causes

When you have studied this chapter, you will understand and be able to describe the main issues surrounding the causes of ADHD and autism.

Key Points

- The causes of ADHD and autism are not entirely known, and there are likely to be multiple causes and complex interactions.
- Many theories have been proposed to account for ADHD and autism.
- There is reliable evidence for a genetic component and evidence of structural and functional brain abnormality.
- Genetic research provides the best potential for understanding the underlying causes.

Aetiology: Theories and Causes

Causation

Perhaps the most significant question is, 'Why do children's developmental conditions occur?', and this may be the hardest question to answer. Both autism and ADHD are not caused by any one thing that we can definitively identify. Frustrating the search for answers is that both autism and ADHD are not singular disorders, so there cannot be a simple response to this question. It is likely that the reply to the central question is that there are many different causes. Psychological research into autism and ADHD that uses large samples of diagnosed individuals in group designs, and generalises from these, may well be 'washing out' results by combining individuals on the basis that they have a similar diagnosis. If there are different routes into these conditions, we must identify them if we are looking for underlying causes, rather than search for general causes of all instances of ADHD and autism. For these reasons, it is doubtful we will ever have a general theory of either autism or ADHD.

Many people are satisfied to stay at the descriptive level of examination when considering both the autism spectrum and the subtypes of ADHD. However, a deeper understanding and appreciation of some of the background theory of these conditions can help to contextualise the outward behaviours seen in people with a diagnosis.

It is true that understanding the possible causes may not contribute to remediating the most troubling of challenges faced by individuals with these conditions, but it is needed if scientific advancements in identification and treatment are to be made. In short, we try to identify the causes of developmental conditions to be best able to progress our understanding of the behaviours that ultimately arise because of them.

When we consider the underlying causes of a condition at the psychological level, we should realise that we use the term 'theory' in a convenient way. Psychological theories in most senses are not theories about cause and effect; they do not set up scientific hypotheses to test root causes of disorders. In this sense, we use 'theory' to describe a set of ideas about a psychological principle or phenomenon; they are explanatory and help us to understand the expression of a condition. Even so, in the scientific sense, we cannot prove a hypothesis, only discard or remove those we know not to be true and move towards a better understanding of possible causes. We seek to present ideas based on the available evidence and welcome challenges to these, and, considering critique, we try to generate better ideas.

In Psychology, like many other disciplines, complex ideas are usually presented as models and theories to be critiqued, rather than as absolute truth. As time passes, scientific knowledge is built up, and we refine ideas, progressing to better understanding. Our awareness of the causes of autism, ADHD and childhood developmental conditions has become better considering new methods, theories and technologies, but they are always speculative. However, these psychological ideas about developmental conditions, which are mostly first diagnosed in childhood, often exist to comprehend behaviour directly and are supported by knowledge of biological and genetic processes – modern-day Psychology is inseparable from these other disciplines.

'Experts' assume each level of enquiry and explanation in different ways to view any given condition. For example, family doctors and Psychiatrists may use a physiological or biological framework, whereas Psychologists and teachers may use another. Professionals, including theorists and researchers, asking fundamental questions about the origins of clinical conditions, vary in the way they perceive and understand those conditions, in keeping with their preoccupations, education and training. There is a risk that each authority may tend to view a condition only through the lens of their own expertise and training.

Differing viewpoints are most apparent in the language that professionals use and their assumptions about general principles of cause-effect or disease–symptom relationships or of the emergent behaviours that arise because of multifaceted developmental disorders. There are many ways of describing the multiple systems of human functioning, for example, the biological, emotional, psychological and social, but rarely is a condition viewed holistically, considering all these levels of explanation.

It can be hard to get a full understanding of distinct disciplines and bodies of research. This book, for example, offers mainly the psychological view of the individual in relation to ADHD and the autism spectrum. The key skill is to know what level of enquiry or explanation to use at any given time and, most importantly, to know how it relates to others. If you are visiting a GP - be on the look-out for the medical perspective; an Educational Psychologist – the cognitive approach; a Social Worker – the social; a school SENCo/SENDCo – the educational. They may all talk about the same child using very different styles of language and terminology, and each may have a different set of assumptions and biases.

It is true to say that one does not need a detailed theoretical understanding of ADHD or autism to accept and appreciate people with these conditions, but it can help. Acceptance and understanding can result from knowledge about underlying causes. Most people have heard of both ADHD and autism, but further understanding of these conditions and what causes them is needed. More importantly, general understanding of the way they affect people's everyday lives is required.

This public lack of understanding is being addressed by the campaign work of advocacy groups that support and represent people with these complex conditions, their families and those that care for them. Two such groups are:

- The ADHD Foundation – www.adhdfoundation.org.uk
- The National Autistic Society – www.autism.org.uk

Understanding the Causes of ADHD

ADHD is a developmental disability with a childhood onset that typically results in a chronic and pervasive pattern of impairment in school, social and/or work domains and often in daily adaptive functioning. One way of thinking about ADHD is as several conditions clustered into a large diagnostic group of symptoms that frequently occur together. There is support for the notion that ADHD is, in fact, several separate conditions (J. Swanson et al., 2000): at least three subtypes affecting inattention and hyperactivity-impulsivity, of probable separate genetic origin involving the dopamine and noradrenaline (norepinephrine) pathways of the brain that oversee learning and motor control.

The core issues that a person diagnosed with ADHD faces originate with problems of the fine-tuning in the normal brain. Neurological evidence leads to the suggestion that there are imbalances in neurotransmitters (the chemical messengers) in parts of the brain responsible for self-monitoring. This idea is a plausible and appealing way to frame the underlying causes of ADHD, but, in practice, this is hard to verify and is not very specific; this can be said of almost any brain-based condition. For example, psychophysiological explanations of ADHD can tell us about the structure (size and shape) and function (information processing) of the typical and atypical brain under certain conditions but are hardly a good way to determine the motivations for the behaviours of a child with ADHD in the school classroom.

ADHD is characterised by three broad groupings of symptoms:

i)   Poor attention.
ii)   High levels of hyperactivity and impulsivity.
iii)   Combinations of these existing together.

ADHD is most apparent at the behavioural level; in this sense, some researchers refer to it as an 'externalising' condition. The observable symptoms are apparent and disruptive to others. In contrast, autism can be viewed as 'internalising'; there are fewer immediately visible markers for the observer to note. The person with autism consumes less of the world of those around them and often seems to be more absorbed in their own behaviour than that of others. However, for the child diagnosed with ADHD or Hyperkinetic Disorder, their presence is immediately felt and is often disruptive to those around them.

The causes of ADHD are not fully known and are likely to have multiple causes and complex interactions. As ADHD includes some very different characteristics, it is to be expected that there will be a number of contributory factors (Empson, 2015). Just as ADHD can manifest in a variety of ways, there are likely to be many causes of ADHD.

This ambiguity of the aetiology or causes for ADHD has led to much speculation about what the underlying causes of the condition are, and this, in turn, may have contributed to the poor public understanding of the condition. There is much work to be done in furthering the public understanding of ADHD and removing the notion that it is in some way causally related to poor parenting or malicious intent on the child's part. ADHD is a neurological condition that affects the course of a child's development and their everyday functioning. This problem with identifying the exact causes has given rise to all manner of explanations for ADHD.

The problem with inhibiting unplanned responses and stopping oneself from going down an automatic path of behaviour is often a core factor in ADHD. This may be one of the first hints that ADHD may have something to do with the problem of inhibiting a response. For example, if the child is in class and there is a window close by and a car goes by, making a loud noise, they may stop attending to the teacher and be up out of their seat at the window and now engaged in a different task. Filtering-out distractions can be extremely difficult for the child with ADHD.

ADHD is mainly a problem with inhibiting certain undesirable behaviours. To maintain the desired behaviour is to stay on task, to selectively attend to the school work and to keep attention on it. For example, the car passing by a window needs to be actively and automatically inhibited at some level of processing; the child needs to resist the temptation to set shift, to maintain the current attentional set and to recognise the vehicle passing but not let it stop the current task. These are complex behavioural activities that require active inhibitory processes that we take for granted but are extremely demanding for the child with ADHD. Children with ADHD may rely on many separate and yet interacting brain processes to unconsciously work together to inhibit the distraction.

A core problem for the child with ADHD is the active inhibition of a 'prepotent' response for which there is immediate reinforcement (positive or negative), rather than as a problem of attention. These problems, coupled with behavioural over-activity and impulsiveness in decision making, can create a *perfect storm* of disruption for the child with the combined form of ADHD. As Russell Barkley states in his classic text on the topic, ADHD is not a "...disorder of knowing what to do, but a disorder of doing what one knows" (1997, p. 16).

There are huge demands placed on children in the everyday school classroom; they must conform much more so than in adulthood. They are required to sit still, to be quiet at times and to solely focus their attention on one teacher talking about things they may not be inclined to learn. Expectations of behaviour at school vary widely, but for children with ADHD, it can be an agonising task. These children typically have a poor ability to persist with a sequence of activities and to engage in tedious or tasks that they find boring and that require sustained mental effort.

Risk Factors for ADHD

Prenatal and perinatal risks, psychosocial factors, and environmental toxins have all been considered as potential risk factors for ADHD. Many of the same risk factors as seen in autism apply to the considerations of ADHD, especially those surrounding heritability. Although the genetic risks implicated in ADHD tend to have small effect sizes, they are reported to increase the risk of many other types of psychopathology. Consequently, these risk factors are not unique to ADHD and cannot be used for prediction, genetic testing or diagnostic purposes beyond what is predicted by family history (Thapar et al., 2013). It is known that both inherited and non-inherited factors contribute to the risk of having ADHD and that their effects are interdependent; as such, no single risk factor explains ADHD.

Biological Considerations of ADHD

The deficits in 'executive function' abilities (the control centre of the brain) of children with ADHD chiefly arise from brain development. According to Russell Barkley (2013, 1997b), ADHD is caused by multiple biological causes and not social factors such as parenting. Executive function abilities are related to the frontal lobe region of the brain, and this is thought to be 2–3 years delayed in children with ADHD. The result of this delayed maturation and under-regulation, coupled with an early developing primary motor cortex (the part of the brain that controls voluntary movement), is ultimately ADHD.

ADHD is a profoundly genetic condition; about 25–35 percent of siblings have the condition, and this rises to 78-92 percent in identical twins with a high proportion of parents demonstrating the symptoms yet remaining undiagnosed. Twin studies show that there is no contribution of the role of parenting to the existence of the condition, although parental training interventions are valuable to help in managing children's behaviour. Although ADHD is a disorder of executive function, issues of heredity, neurobiology, environment and society all play an essential part in understanding it.

About 10–15 percent of ADHD arises because of prenatal injuries to the development of the prefrontal cortex (Barkley, 2000). About 3–5 percent of ADHD arises because of postnatal brain damage from, for example, trauma (head injury) or streptococcal infections. These acquired cases of ADHD happen mainly in boys, as the male brain is more prone to injury prenatally and postnatally than the female brain. However, overwhelmingly, most instances of ADHD are heritable; in these cases, the affected brain regions are reported to be about 3–10 percent smaller, giving rise to the condition.

The regions of the brain implicated in ADHD are the orbital prefrontal cortex, the basal ganglia, the cerebellum, the anterior cingulate cortex and the corpus callosum. According to Barkley, the size of these regions is directly related to the severity of ADHD. However, the structural brain differences (size and shape) in children with ADHD are not sufficiently smaller to do reliable diagnostic scanning, and by around the age of 16–18 years, the size of the regions normalises but the functioning remains delayed.

Psychological Considerations of ADHD

Recently, genetic research has started to show the best potential for understanding the underlying aetiology of ADHD. Psychological explanations can explain the expression of the largely underlying genetic heritance of the condition, which affects brain development and, in turn, psychological function.

Russell Barkley (1997a, 2014) has developed one of the leading psychological theories of ADHD. His ideas about the contribution of self-regulation (response inhibition) and executive dysfunction have led to greater understanding of the condition and ultimately the role of genetic factors.

For Barkley, the capacity for regulating self-control is neuro-genetic and not social; it is not a learnt ability. The inability to direct behaviour towards the self comes from impairments in executive abilities that are shaped and affected by social considerations but are not caused by them. He cites a series of central 'executive abilities' that are delayed in children with ADHD. Self-regulation is the first and most crucial executive ability affected in ADHD. Waiting for a task to finish, inhibiting or building in a pause, and self-regulating one's behaviour are critical skills that affect all other abilities and are grossly affected in children with ADHD. Likewise, the capacity to use and remember visual mental imagery to give foresight is affected. Internalised speech (private speech) is affected too. This ability is used to regulate behaviour and is apparent in young children as they talk through activities to themselves; in later years, this becomes internalised. Similarly, the capacity to self-motivate, to delay gratification for a later reward and to manage one's emotions are affected. Finally, planning and problem-solving are affected, so the ability to simulate multiple possible solutions to a problem before acting on one is impaired.

> 'Response inhibition' is the "...ability to withhold a cognitive or behavioural impulse that may be inaccurate or maladaptive."
>
> (Mary Solanto in Barkley 2014, p. 257)

Most people with ADHD have no difficulties concentrating when they are doing something that interests them, whether it is educational or for entertainment. The ability to 'hyperfocus', to stay intensely on task for a long time, is a common trait in children with ADHD and suggests that the condition is not one purely of attentional dysfunction. This phenomenon is often observed in children with ADHD who sometimes can play intense video games for prolonged periods of time. Unlike in the classroom or doing homework, video games continually reward and reinforce engagement; the rules are consistent, and engagement is controllable. They can maintain their focus for hours because the rewards are concrete, frequent and immediate, rather than abstract, sparse and delayed.

Barkley's conceptualisation of ADHD is one where neuropsychological impairment leads to deficits in executive functions, self-regulation, and behavioural or 'response inhibition' (Barkley, 1997a, 2014). Self-regulation is the ability to inhibit; to delay; to separate thought from feeling, and to consider an experience and change perspective. The ability to consider alternative responses, choose a response and act successfully towards a goal gives a person the ability to negotiate life automatically and to track cues appropriately. Poor self-regulation leads to impulsive, 'cue-less' behaviour that is inconsistent and unpredictable. The person with ADHD continually rides an emotional roller coaster and has problems with automatic behaviour.

The markers of ADHD may well be the psychological manifestations of an underlying delay in brain development, but to say that there is a single cause of ADHD would be misleading. The psychological level of enquiry gives us insights into possible ways that the condition can present itself. However, ADHD, like autism, exists on a continuum of impairment that differs in both its severity and its presentation.

Other Suggested Causes of ADHD

There have been many other theories of ADHD proposed, including animal and biomedical models, many of these are outside the field of Psychology and thus are mainly outside the remit of this book. Other possible causes of ADHD that have been suggested with differing degrees of support are, for example, lead ingestion; stress; emotional problems; allergies; lack of essential fatty acids; free radicals; and vitamin deficiency. These are not dissimilar to those proposed causes of autism, most often lacking in empirical support, that have been suggested and are often popularised by the media from time to time.

Scepticism towards ADHD

Although ADHD is one of the most frequently occurring and well-researched conditions of childhood, it is also one of the most controversial and misunderstood of all psychiatric diagnoses. "No mental disability this decade has been assailed by as much criticism, scepticism and flat out mockery as ADHD", said Mathew Cohen, president of Children and Adults with Attention Deficit Disorder (CHADD) (Kennedy, 2009, p. 1)

Angered by the increasing negative media portrayal of ADHD, a group of nearly 80 Psychiatrists and Psychologists led by Russell Barkley published a very public Consensus Statement on the science, diagnosis and treatment of ADHD (2002). In this scathing attack on the suggestion that 'ADHD does not exist', Barkley and colleagues cited mounting evidence of the neurological and genetic contributions to the disorder. They stressed that ADHD is not a benign disorder and can cause 'devastating problems' for those it afflicts, yet studies indicate that most people with the disorder are not receiving treatment.

In a now-classic article, two British Psychiatrists with profoundly opposing views, Sami Timimi and Eric Taylor, were featured in the British Journal of Psychiatry (Timimi & Taylor, 2004). Controversially, Timimi suggested that ADHD can be best understood as a cultural construct; that it is a creation of society itself and unnecessarily over-diagnosed. Taylor suggested the opposite: that ADHD is under-diagnosed, under-detected, and a genuine and debilitating medical condition. Each researcher continues to publish compelling arguments for their respective viewpoints, and the debate continues to illuminate both the validity of diagnostic psychopathology and the importance of considering the efficacy and ethics of the psychiatric assessment and treatment of children.

ADHD is one of the most researched psychiatric diagnoses, yet uncertainty over the validity of the condition continues to polarise public opinion. Rafalovich (2005) found that many doctors are no more confident in the diagnosis and treatment of ADHD than many parents are. The uncertainty of some about the ADHD diagnosis and treatment is likely due to the heterogeneity of the disorder, the perceived controversy regarding the misuse of stimulant medications and frequent misrepresentation in the media.

Understanding the Causes of Autism

The epidemiological data currently available on the prevalence and distribution of autism suggests that about 1 percent of the UK population has an autism spectrum condition, which is around a twentyfold increase in the 50 years since the first study to record its prevalence. However, current methods for recording the instances of autism in the community (diagnosed or undiagnosed) are based on estimates and are likely to change further, given the continual reclassification of the condition in the diagnostic manuals.

Risk Factors for Autism

We know about some of the possible causes of autism but not the whole story. Most scientists agree that a genetic risk factor can make a person more likely to develop autism.

Several well-documented risk factors increase the chance of a child being born with an autism spectrum condition. Twin studies have demonstrated that genetic heritability is the most significant contributor to having autism. There is a much higher concordance of autism in identical twins than in non-identical twins or siblings.

The sex of the child is also associated with autism frequency, with boys being up to three times more likely to have autism than girls are. The sex difference, however, may be to do with vulnerabilities of the male brain during development in pregnancy, rather than genetics. Likewise, the environment may also be a contributory risk factor for autism. Acquired infections during pregnancy, pesticides and smoking are all possible risk factors. Likewise, the age of the mother is a consideration too. Mothers over 40 years old have about a 50 percent increased chance of having a child with autism than mothers between the ages of 20 and 29 years old. Paternal age, contributing to poorer sperm quality, is also a possible contributory factor to a higher chance of having a child with autism. These risk factors are not unique to autism and are difficult to generalise from. Perinatal risk factors, around the time of birth itself, have also been documented, such as prolonged labour, stress and lack of oxygen in birth.

For more information, see https://www.cdc.gov/ncbddd/autism/features/keyfindings-risk-factors.html.

Biological Considerations of Autism

There are many biological theories of autism, and these are best viewed alongside psychological theories to provide a representation of the likely cause and manifestation of behaviours in autism.

There is about 60–95 percent concordance in autism between monozygotic (identical) twins; meaning that if you share identical genes with someone with autism, you are likely to have autism yourself. This figure drops to around 5–10 percent in dizygotic (fraternal) twins, who do not share identical genes, and around 2–8 percent in non-twin siblings. Therefore, we know with reliably that genes play a dominant role in the causes of autism. However, the exact genetic underpinnings of autism remain unknown in more than 80 percent of cases (Kanduri et al., 2016). It is doubtful that there is a single gene responsible for autism; a 'single-hit' hypothesis has been ruled out for some time.

It is possible for there to be genetic causes of autism that are not a result of inherited genes from parents. Damage, of mostly unknown origin, or mutations to the sperm or egg, mainly to the egg (as it contributes the most cellular structure), can result in vulnerability to autism. Altered gene expression may lead to abnormal brain development, resulting in autism. It is speculated that this epigenetic hypothesis, arising from non-genetic influences on gene expression, may account for the effect of environmental toxins on gene expression and regulation, and this idea has gained much attention in recent years. This idea does give rise to the possibility of potential epigenetic therapies targeting affected genes, but this research is not established (Mehler & Purpura, 2009). Though in their early stages, studies of epigenetic change in autism have the potential to increase our understanding of the causes of the condition (Loke, Hannan, & Craig, 2015).

It may be the case that although individuals have a genetic vulnerability to developing autism, it is possible that several environmental triggers are also needed. The 'multi-hit' hypothesis suggests that there are multiple contributing factors combined that lead to autism. These many combined paths result in the disturbance of brain development. For example, contributing factors may be chemical, genetic or autoimmune in nature. This idea has some credibility, given that autism, like ADHD, is defined by combinations of symptoms, rather than a single underlying identifying cause.

Damage to the foetus from exposure to chemicals in utero has been suggested as a possible cause of autism in some circumstances. Toxicology theories of autism are wide-ranging, but there is increasing evidence of this pathway that warrants further investigation.

Some parents report that their children do not exhibit recognisable symptoms of autism until 15–30 months or may show a regression around this time, for example losing language or social skills – the so-called 'autism regression' reported in some children. This regression may lead parents to suspect that certain environmental factors are responsible for autism, and there is controversy and speculation around this issue.

Other hypotheses have been suggested, such as the role of autoimmune disease in pregnancy, where the mother's antibodies cause inflammation in the foetal brain. Likewise, certain pro-inflammatory conditions, such as rheumatoid arthritis and coeliac disease, have been linked to autism, yet evidence of a general causal relationship is still to be established.

Psychological Considerations of Autism

The biological basis of autism has been accepted for many years, and progress is being made on further specifying this. However, the study of the behavioural and underlying cognitive deficits in autism has advanced ahead of the study of the underlying brain abnormalities and genetic mechanisms (Hill & Frith, 2003). Psychological research and areas such as developmental cognitive neuroscience help us to further our understanding of autism.

Three major cognitive theories have dominated psychological investigation into autism (Rajendran & Mitchell, 2007). These are: i) 'theory-of-mind' deficit theory, which involves social and communication impairments; ii) executive function deficit theory, which seeks to explore stereotyped behaviour and narrow interests; and iii) weak central coherence theory, which suggests that local (rather than global) processing is at the heart of this condition. As such, we examine each briefly here.

Theory-of-Mind Deficit
Early in the study of autism, the research identified that individuals on the spectrum fail to attribute mental states to themselves and others (Premack & Woodruff, 1978). This appears as an inability to 'mentalise'

or a failure to consider other people's mental states – a so-called 'theory-of-mind' deficit. Tasks exploring these abilities in children with autism suggest a lack of understanding that people's actions are based on their own beliefs, even when those beliefs deviate from what the child knows to be true.

Early theorising used evidence from 'false-belief' tests to show that failure in understanding the minds of others is a core deficit in people with autism (Baron-Cohen, Leslie, & Frith, 1985; Wimmer & Perner, 1983). Although these studies were widely replicated (e.g., Perner, Frith, Leslie, & Leekam, 1989), it was shown that about 20 percent of people with autism passed this type of test (Happé, 1994). Subsequently, the theory-of-mind deficit notion of autism was modified by embracing the idea that these difficulties in people with autism were delayed, rather than deficient. A key theorist was Simon Baron-Cohen, who used a more-difficult second-order false-belief task (e.g. "I think he thinks she thinks") and showed that 90 percent of typically developing children, but none of the children with autism he tested, passed (1989). Baron-Cohen concluded that because individuals with autism could not pass a second-order task, they did not have a fully formed 'representational theory of mind'. Subsequently, Bowler (1992) challenged the idea that theory-of-mind development was delayed at all in autism, finding that 73 percent of young adults with Asperger's Syndrome could pass second-order false-belief tasks.

Although the 'theory-of-mind deficit hypothesis' is no longer considered to be a credible causal theory of autism, in historical terms it brought Developmental Psychology into mainstream autism research. These explanations show a long history of academic experimentation around the problems faced by people on the autistic spectrum and focus largely on the impairments in socialisation, imagination and communication demonstrated by individuals with autism. We know today that people's abilities are wide-ranging and that theory-of-mind problems are not unique to people on the autism spectrum. Children with autism generally show evidence of the development of theory-of-mind abilities at around 4–5 years of age – significantly later than typically developing children.

Although initially thought of as a core deficit of autism and by some as a cause of many of the features of autism, researchers have now come to understand theory-of-mind difficulties as arising because of the features of autism, rather than as a cause of autism itself. Children with autism frequently display many symptoms that are not specific to the condition, such as language impairment, stereotyped behaviour and lower intelligence. Because of this, Happé (1994) argued that it is important for theories of autism to focus on the features that are specific to autism.

Executive Dysfunction

Executive function refers to the brain processes underlying the control of behaviours, such as working memory, planning, inhibitory control and attentional set shifting. The executive dysfunction theory of autism suggests that deficits in these abilities underlie the cognitive impairments found in children with autism (Hughes, Russell, & Robbins, 1994; Ozonoff, Pennington, & Rogers, 1991).

The disruption of executive processes results in individuals with autism displaying difficulties in new or ambiguous situations but no impairment on well-learnt or routine tasks and may explain their so-called stereotyped behaviours and narrow interests. This profile is evidenced by individuals with autism performing poorly on tests of executive function despite being able to pass theory-of-mind tasks. Early research by Hughes and Russell (1993) argued that 'on-line' executive control is necessary to pass false-belief tasks; failure of theory-of-mind tasks may just be because the demands on the capacity of the processes in these are too high.

Although these ideas moved us closer to a *modular* brain-based conceptualisation of the possible causes of autism, this theory does lack discriminative validity. The executive impairments that are seen in autism also appear in some other developmental disorders, for example, ADHD, Tourette's Syndrome and Conduct Disorder. It is not possible to know if executive impairments are the primary cause of the disorder or appear later and are consequences of autism.

Weak Central Coherence

The 'weak central coherence' hypothesis of autism suggests that there is a cognitive bias towards local rather than global information processing. Typically-developing (neurotypical) people have the tendency to pull information together, process it in context and draw out the meaning, often at the expense of details. However, it is suggested that people with autism have weak central coherence and attend to and remember details, rather than global form or meaning (Happé, 2013).

In short, there is a tendency to attend to the constituent parts or fine detail of something, rather than to experience it as a whole. This processing bias can be considered a cognitive style rather than an impairment and as such offers a view of autism that is refreshing and not characterised by impairment.

For example, people with autism tend not to succumb to visual illusions (Happé, 1996) but do fail to use context in reading (Happé, 1995). The theory proposes that in the typical cognitive system, something exists that enables the processing of incoming information in context for global meaning; this helps us to make sense of the world (Hill & Frith, 2003). In people with autism, this cognitive style is different and can explain both the deficits found in autism and the strengths exhibited by individuals with autism.

The ability to detach from context and process fine detail is an advantage in many visuospatial tasks. For example, people with autism tend to have superior performance on tasks where they are asked to identify embedded figures within a complex picture or on block design tasks, where the ability to process unique features coupled with the poor processing of similar features is an advantage.

If children with autism excel at processing stimuli without reference to context, this predicts that they would be unable to understand linguistic ambiguities, such as words or sentences with dual meanings. In classic reading research, Frith and Snowling (1983) showed that many children with autism only demonstrated reading failure when it was necessary for them to take context into account.

Pragmatic language impairments are common to several developmental conditions (e.g. ADHD and autism) where the basics of language and literacy may be intact, but the ability to use language socially is impaired (Bignell & Cain, 2007; Bishop in Bishop & Leonard, 2014). These difficulties may be linked to weak coherence, theory-of-mind deficit or executive dysfunction, but the empirical validity of these in explaining pragmatic language impairment in autism may be limited (Martin & McDonald, 2003). In light of changes to the diagnosis of autism, a new clinical disorder, Social (Pragmatic) Communication Disorder, was added to the Neurodevelopmental Disorders section of DSM-5 (Baird & Norbury, 2015).

Researcher Kate Plaisted points out that a number of studies show that individuals with autism are able to attend selectively to either the global or local level of processing when directed to do so, but in tasks of divided attention, they display a preference to process at the local level (Plaisted in Burack, Charman, Yirmiya, & Zelazo, 2001). She suggests that individuals with autism have difficulty making sense of the world because of an impaired ability to process the similar features between stimuli or situations, which hinders the transfer of learning from one situation to another. These ideas may explain the reduced ability to generalise learning seen in individuals with autism.

Other Suggested Causes of Autism

Numerous less-established ideas about autism have been proposed in recent years, many having little or no support for them, while others do provide some confirmation in the published academic literature. These include, for example, allergies; 'leaky gut' (intestine problems); food intolerances; specific environmental toxins; and nutritional/vitamin deficiency.

Further research is needed to establish the credibility of many of these ideas. Other more-controversial ideas, such as the suggestion that poor parenting, or mercury in vaccines (now generally no longer used), is responsible for autism hold little to no scientific credibility and are generally considered to be distracting from our understanding of autism.

The Extreme Male Brain

In his book, *The Essential Difference*, leading theorist and researcher Simon Baron-Cohen (2003) outlines what he calls the 'Extreme Male Brain'. He characterises autism as one end of a continuum of the 'systemising–empathising' scale. Systemising is the drive to analyse or construct a system: the rules or laws that govern that system to predict how it will behave. Empathising is different: it is about being able to imagine what someone else is thinking or feeling and having an emotional response to the other person's feelings.

For Baron-Cohen, males tend to have a stronger drive to systemise and females have a stronger drive to empathise. He suggests that people on the autism spectrum show an exaggeration of the male profile. Theory of mind is part of empathy, so people at the opposite systemising end show problems with this ability.

Baron-Cohen's ideas hold much ground in describing the differences seen in people on the autism spectrum, both their strengths and weaknesses. However, there is a risk that these ideas may over-represent individuals with autism at the milder end of the continuum and under-represent those many people with autism who show significant intellectual disabilities but no speech disabilities (Buchen, 2011).

The causes of both autism and ADHD are reported to be mostly genetic and highly heritable and can be understood through a biological underpinning with a psychological manifestation. They are conditions that are diagnosed mainly by observed characteristics and behaviour, rather than their causes, and as such are defined by groups of symptoms that frequently occur together to form agreed-upon psychiatric classifications. These conditions are likely to be polygenetic in nature, having no single underlying cause.

We will look at coexisting conditions that often go alongside autism and ADHD in more detail in Chapter 6.

Resources

For more information about autism, visit the National Autistic Society at their website:

www.autism.org.uk.

For more information about ADHD and related conditions, visit the ADHD Foundation at their website:

www.adhdfoundation.org.uk.

If you would like to consider taking part in research studies about autism and ADHD, please visit www.ASDresearch.org to register your interest.

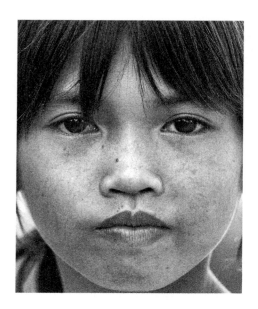

Chapter 6 – Comorbidity: Coexisting Conditions

When you have studied this chapter, you will understand and be able to describe the main issues surrounding comorbidity in autism and ADHD in detail.

Key Points

- Comorbidity is common in developmental disorders, and many clinical conditions often occur alongside both ADHD and autism.
- There is also a high overlap between the symptoms of ADHD and autism.
- Most research studies exclude cases of autism from studies on ADHD and vice versa.
- The high comorbidity with other conditions may suggest a common root or represent difficulties with current classification systems or selection bias in comorbidity research.
- Interactions between clinical conditions have implications for

differential diagnoses, assessment and treatment.

What is Comorbidity?

Comorbidity is the presence of one or more psychiatric diagnoses in addition to a primary diagnosis. Quite simply, it is the "co-occurrence of different diseases in the same individual" (Blashfield, 1990, p. 61). Comorbidity with other clinical disorders is to be expected in autism (Gillberg & Billstedt, 2000). Research into the inherited and genetic contributions to ADHD suggests a substantial overlap with autism (Thapar et al., 2013).

There exist distinct types of comorbidity, according to First (2005):

i)   Where there are clinically distinct entities occurring together.
ii)   Where there is artefactual comorbidity, a by-product of the diagnostic criteria.
iii)   False comorbidity.

As First describes:

"It is important to understand that comorbidity in psychiatry does not imply the presence of multiple diseases or dysfunctions but rather reflects our current inability to apply... a single diagnosis to account for all symptoms."

(First, 2005, p. 1).

Diagnostic psychiatric categories mainly act to bring together sets of behaviours, without any indication of the underlying causes. Comorbidities are mostly defined by the co-presence of another diagnostic category, rather than by individual symptoms, for example, ADHD and Major Depressive Disorder. However, it is also possible to specify comorbidity in a less rigid way at the symptom level, for example, hyperactivity and anxiety. The use of fixed diagnostic categories or more-expressive symptom descriptors largely depends on why one is communicating such information.

Historically, depending on which diagnostic manual was consulted, the categories of ADHD and autism existed alongside other closely related conditions. For example, ADHD was listed alongside conditions like Conduct Disorder and Oppositional Defiant Disorder in the DSM-IV-TR (diagnostic manual) (American Psychiatric Association, 2000). Likewise, autism was included as a Pervasive Developmental Disorder alongside Rett's Disorder, Childhood Disintegrative Disorder and a separate category: Asperger's Disorder, which is now formally included as part of Autism Spectrum Disorder.

In the diagnostic manual versions before DSM-5, autism and ADHD were mutually exclusive: it was not possible to diagnose both concurrently. The exclusion criteria restricted a dual diagnosis of these conditions. However, there was little empirical evidence demonstrating that the hierarchy imposed by such exclusion criteria was meaningful (Slade & Andrews, 2002). In the latest revision of the diagnostic manual (DSM-5, American Psychiatric Association, 2013), individuals can be diagnosed with both autism and ADHD at the same time.

Comorbidity in ADHD

As many as one-third of children diagnosed with ADHD also have a coexisting diagnosed condition. The symptoms of ADHD frequently overlap with symptoms of other related disorders. Common coexisting conditions in children with ADHD include anxiety disorders and disorders of mood, conduct, learning, motor control, social communication and reading.

In adults, ADHD often is reported to occur in people who also have Personality Disorder, Bipolar Disorder, Obsessive-Compulsive Disorder and substance misuse (National Institute for Health and Care Excellence, 2013b). Notably, learning disabilities also occur in about 25 percent of children with ADHD, especially receptive language problems (comprehension and understanding) and expressive language problems (written output and speech).

A wide variety of problems coexist alongside ADHD (Taylor, 2011). A diagnosis of ADHD is almost always an indication that there will be other difficulties, even if they are undiagnosed. For example, comorbidity between ADHD and language, reading and speech disorders occurs so regularly that it has led to a general acceptance of the overlap between communication disorders and behaviour disorders (Tomblin & Mueller, 2012). Even in non-diagnosed samples of children, poor attention and elevated levels of hyperactivity are consistently associated with pragmatic language weaknesses (Bignell & Cain, 2007).

However, ADHD is wide-ranging and likely to have multiple causes. According to Thomas Brown, ADHD is not just one of many different psychiatric disorders:

> "It is a foundational disorder that substantially increases a person's risk of experiencing additional cognitive, emotional, or behavior disorders across the lifespan".
>
> (Brown, 2009, p. 13).

More than any other psychiatric diagnoses, ADHD tends to appear in combination with other conditions. For example, in the famous large-scale 'MTA study', 70 percent of children with ADHD met the full diagnostic criteria for at least one other psychiatric disorder (Jensen et al., 2001)

Comorbidity in Autism

When a person has autism, there is a high probability that they will have other conditions. Comorbid disorders occur in around 70 percent of individuals with autism, and these problems can substantially affect the person's quality of life and that of their families or carers, leading to social vulnerability (NICE, 2014).

A large number of medical conditions, psychiatric disorders and behavioural and motor dyscontrol symptoms are associated with autism and Asperger's Syndrome (Gillberg & Billstedt, 2000). These include, most frequently, ADHD but also Depression, Anxiety, Tourette's Syndrome, Personality Disorders, Selective Mutism, Eating Disorders, Substance Use Disorders and Sleep Disorders. The list is similar to that of the comorbidities seen in ADHD.

Comorbidity is to be expected in autism, with about 50 percent of people with autism also have an intellectual disability (Learning Disability) (Gillberg & Billstedt, 2000). Frequently people with autism also have a sensitivity to light, sound, touch, smell, taste and/or balance problems. As well as other psychological conditions, physical conditions are also frequently reported alongside autism. Commonly occurring medical conditions that are sometimes reported alongside autism are Tuberous Sclerosis, Fragile X, Rett's Syndrome and brain damage following Encephalitis. It is important that the diagnostic assessment process includes a full physical health check by a medical practitioner.

Some specific patterns of disabilities and/or behaviour that can be seen in some people with autism have named them as separate syndromes. For example, 'Semantic-Pragmatic Disorder' is a term sometimes still used to describe people with perserved grammatical language but a lack of ability to use language in a socially appropriate manner. Increasingly the diagnosis of Social (pragmatic) Communication Disorder is used to describe some people who would have otherwise attracted a diagnosis of Autism.

More recently a new category, Pathological Demand Avoidance (PDA), is being used by some to describe people who show avoidance of everyday tasks and can show manipulative, socially inappropriate, in some cases aggressive, behaviour. With some diagnoses, the relationship to autism is ambiguous. These conditions are like autism in some respects, but increased understanding of autism and related conditions is allowing us to make tighter distinctions between diagnostic categories, where before we may have relied on less-specific categorisation. Future editions of the diagnostic manuals, informed by research, will lead to new categories that help provide more tailored and directed support. Many of these may well better describe some people who are currently diagnosed with autism.

The National Autistic Society lists information about the use and misuse of diagnostic labels in autism here: www.autism.org.uk/labels.

Similarities Between Autism and Other Conditions

The relationship between Obsessive Compulsive Disorder (OCD) and autism highlights a few of the inherent problems of comorbidity and differential diagnosis in the fields of Psychology and Psychiatry. The obsessions of people diagnosed with OCD may be mistaken for parts of the classic 'triad of impairment' used to descriptive autism. However, the special interests often seen in people with autism are not the same as the 'obsessions' of people with OCD. In autism, thoughts may be rigid and inflexible, but they tend not to be as intrusive as in OCD. The special interests of individuals with autism are not problematic; they are typically pleasurable for the individuals with autism. Typically, in the autistic person, this gathering of a wealth of information about a particular topic is obsessive but not inherently (cognitively) problematic.

The similarity between conditions and the possible overlap of symptoms can be demonstrated if we look at some of the shared features of autism and Schizophrenia. Many of the markers for autism can easily be misinterpreted as signs of Schizophrenia. For example, a person with autism may often have or appear to have disorganised thinking; they can focus on an inner life or make-believe world and sometimes speak thoughts out loud. Likewise, people with autism can often produce fantastic stories, and these can be similar to the delusions or complex visual hallucinations experienced by people with Schizophrenia. Moreover, thoughts described concretely may sound like an auditory hallucination to others, and there can appear to be a similarity between the two conditions. Early studies suggested an association between Schizophrenia and autism; for example, Leo Kanner, one of the first people to identify autism, believed that 'early infantile autism' would not have to be separated from 'the schizophrenias' (Kanner, 1949).

Considerations of Comorbidity

It seems likely that issues of comorbidity do have important implications for treatment. It is not clear as to how the presence of autism symptoms in children with ADHD may impact on responses to medication given for ADHD (Cooper, Martin, Langley, Hamshere, & Thapar, 2013).

One continual problem for the validity of research studies is that investigators often try to reduce the occurrence of comorbidity in their samples. They sometimes do this to reduce the confounding effects of these comorbidities on their results. For example, most genetic studies exclude cases of autism from studies on ADHD and vice versa. Clinical researchers often try to recruit samples of people for their studies with a single primary diagnosis or try to adjust for these factors statistically. For example, recruitment samples may favour individuals with autism but not anxiety, or ADHD without comorbid depression. There is, of course, good reason for employing such methods, but this may have the effect of artificially changing the apparent frequency of comorbidity as it exists in research designs, rather than representing occurring numbers in the community.

ADHD research, where there are distinct diagnostic subtypes, typically attempts to isolate symptoms and investigate the purest form of ADHD possible. However, this is not how the condition manifests in everyday life; seldom do we find ADHD without associated secondary conditions. These exclusion criteria both reinforce the divisions between the subtypes and serve to isolate ADHD from associated comorbidities and secondary characteristics of the condition.

Likewise, in clinical research samples, participants with autism or ADHD are often recruited from assessment centres, clinics, clinicians' practices or places where diagnosed individuals attend for support. These recruited samples are not as they would occur in the community and may lead to artefactual comorbidity from a form of selection bias inherent in many clinic-based research designs. For example, if a person has a single primary diagnosis (i.e. no comorbidity), they are less likely than those with several diagnoses to be present at or involved with the places from which research studies recruit. This is especially true if the individual's condition is not causing problems or affecting other areas of functioning. Selection bias may be one of the reasons that comorbidities appear extremely high across all clinical conditions. Caution may be needed when generalising results from such clinic-based samples to the broader community. Epidemiological or community-based studies are required to show actual rates of comorbidity in the community.

It is important to note that a person with clinical symptoms suggestive of a disorder can be either:

i)   Correctly diagnosed.
ii)   Misdiagnosed.
iii)   Remain undiagnosed.

This last 'undiagnosed' category may account for the most substantial number of people who experience symptoms, either of less severity or which do not present an everyday problem for them if they are sufficiently coping.

The prevalence rates of diagnosed disorders and the reported comorbid ratios between them in the community are not necessarily related to their actual existence but by the degree to which they interfere with the everyday functioning of the people. Psychiatric conditions are chiefly defined by impairment and troublesome symptoms, not by their actual occurrence, which may include desirable symptoms or underlying causes. Likewise, the diagnostic 'status' of a person does not affect the symptoms they experience, which may vary according to internal factors, such as temperament, mood and anxiety, or external factors, such as everyday stressors and changes in their settings or routine.

With conditions such as autism or ADHD, which are mainly assessed by observation of symptoms and clinical case history, the diagnosis or label that is given to a person is not a characteristic of the individual and represents merely a way of describing the group of symptoms a person consistently shows. In this way, the practice of diagnosis can be seen as a convenient way to group people together who show a similar set of indicators for a given condition. This allows clinicians and practitioners to provide more-efficient support structures; it also allows researchers to explore groups of people who show similar symptoms and to make predictions about what may cause these, as well as establish how to remediate them.

Comorbidity, to an extent, is a product of a *categorical* (rather than *dimensional*) diagnostic system that imposes artificial distinctions between clusters of clinical features. The approach mainly derives from Psychiatry, which embraces the 'medical model' of illness. The model replicates traditional physical medicine, where there are commonly direct symptoms of illness and most often an established standard treatment for everyone.

Psychiatrists are physicians and have a medical foundation; it is no surprise then that the leading diagnostic manual for research and diagnosis, published by the American Psychiatric Association (DSM-5, 2013), uses a framework where psychological indicators, markers, characteristics and behaviours that deviate from the norm are viewed as symptoms of diseases and pathologised.

In successive revisions, the DSM-5 has made small steps to move away from a categorical approach to mental illness and related conditions. This, however, is not the only way in which to frame mental illness. A dimensional approach is possible, for diagnoses based on continuous measures of psychopathology that are flexible and fluid and where practitioners treat symptomatically.

As Lopez et al. suggest, "...without satisfactory grounding in aetiology, any diagnostic rubric will remain suboptimal" (2007, p. S6). Following this approach, the diagnoses of the co-occurrence of psychiatric disorders (comorbidity) can be sympathetic to individual differences and diversity among populations and can view that there are likely to be as many paths to psychological health as there are paths to psychological illness.

Overlap of Symptoms in Autism, Asperger's and ADHD

There are significant similarities and overlaps of symptoms in autism, Asperger's and ADHD. At the behavioural level, the indicators of these conditions are often the same. For example, talking and interrupting, poor executive function and planning, and poor turn taking are all indicative of both ADHD and autism; however, the reasons for these are usually not.

Impulsivity, emotional dysregulation and cognitive impairment are all similarly shared between autism and ADHD. Children with both conditions may make naïve remarks, or faux pas, or may be seen to be too honest. Likewise, they often can only be with others on their terms and may be unaware of social conventions or are indifferent to peer pressure. Their strong preferences mean that they are good at some things and poor at others but may act the same with everybody. They may share pragmatic language difficulties and make little language adjustment to fit social context or may take things overly literally. Autism can present with severe hyperactivity and attention problems, and hyperactivity is a common presenting problem in pre-school children with autism.

ADHD and autism are generally described as separate disorders with separate genetic causes. The elevated levels of activity seen in children with ADHD are not a clinical feature of autism. Likewise, the attentional features of autism are different in quality from ADHD. For example, in ADHD, they are mostly externally cued; in autism, these are primarily internally cued by the person's thoughts. Similarly, with ADHD, there is a *lack* of focus (inattention), whereas, with autism, there can be an over-focus on things that the child seems to find interesting.

Several speculative questions remain to be answered within the field:
1) Could ADHD comprise a mixture of other syndromes (e.g. Tourette's, Bipolar, Depression and variants of autism) that all present with some 'ADHD' symptomatology?
2) Could any dopamine/noradrenaline dysfunction syndrome with early onset present as ADHD or a 'shadow syndrome' of ADHD?
3) Could autism, Asperger's and ADHD fall on the same spectrum?

We will look at strategies, interventions and treatment in more detail in Chapter 7.

Resources

For more information about autism, visit the National Autistic Society at their website:

www.autism.org.uk.

For more information about ADHD and related conditions, visit the ADHD Foundation at their website:

www.adhdfoundation.org.uk.

If you would like to consider taking part in research studies about autism and ADHD, please visit www.ASDresearch.org to register your interest.

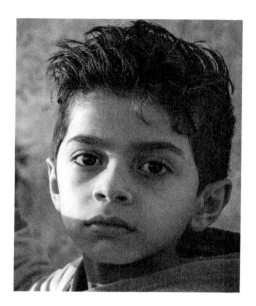

Chapter 7 – Strategies for Care, Interventions and Treatment

When you have studied this chapter, you will understand and be able to describe the main issues surrounding interventions and treatment of ADHD and autism.

Key Points

- There are many different types of interventions for autism and ADHD although not all strategies fit all children.
- Early intervention is considered necessary to change the developmental trajectory of children.
- One treatment can help people with autism is 'Applied Behavioural Analysis' (ABA).
- Psychopharmaceutic medications are effective for most children with ADHD, although some opinions remain divided on its use.
- Conduct problems may hinder the assessment and treatment of ADHD.

- The effectiveness of treatments can depend on the level of severity, communication impairment, comorbid conditions, and associated learning disabilities.

Strategies for Care, Interventions and Treatment

The route to effective treatment is often not straightforward. Parents often must educate themselves as to the best path to treatment and the effectiveness of such. As Diane Kennedy, an author and parent of a child with autism and ADHD, states:

> "...parents of children with these syndromes often must travel alone through a maze of misdiagnoses and ineffective or inappropriate treatments."

> (Kennedy, 2009, p. 11).

There are many different types of interventions for autism and ADHD, although not all strategies fit all children. It can take a long time to find an appropriate and effective strategy to support children. These services are often dependent on the availability of community, school and Local Authority resources.

Early Interventions

Early interventions are essential for improving outcomes for young children with autism (Webb, Jones, Kelly, & Dawson, 2014). However, how and when to intervene are critical questions. These researchers claim that using interventions at an early age when the brain is developing and before autism symptoms have emerged, could significantly alter the developmental course of children at-risk for the disorder. Long-term studies are needed to determine when and how the most-effective early interventions should take place.

Findings suggest that parent training programmes are a valuable strategy for providing support for many pre-school children displaying early signs of ADHD (Jones, Daley, Hutchings, Bywater, & Eames, 2007). Likewise, literature reviews reveal that early intensive behavioural interventions for young children with autism may enhance developmental outcomes (Warren et al., 2011).

The 'Education, Health and Care Plan' and Special Educational Needs

About 70 percent of children with autism are in mainstream education. Likewise, most children with ADHD remain in mainstream schools, where strategies and interventions can be most effective alongside the school curriculum. For many years, it was common for children with ADHD or autism to have a 'Statement of Special Educational Needs', which set out the unique needs of the child and was used as the basis to proceed with strategies of care, interventions and treatment. From 2014, 'statements' began to be phased out and will for some years still be in the process of being replaced with 'Education, Health and Care Plans' (EHC plans / EHCPs). A child must be identified in their school as having special educational needs to have an EHCP.

All children with a diagnosis of autism or ADHD should have an EHCP or an existing Statement of Special Educational Needs, as this informs and underpins treatment and care strategies. The EHCP details a child's educational needs and the support that they require for those needs. It uses a person-centred approach to ensure that children, young people and parents are involved in all aspects of planning and decision making. The complete cycle of EHC needs assessment and EHCP development, from the point when an assessment is requested until the final plan is issued, must take no more than 20 weeks according to Government statutory guidelines. However, the reality in many regions is that this duration is often exceeded and there can be lengthy delays in receiving an assessment.

Published in 2015, the *Special Educational Needs and Disability Code of Practice: 0 to 25 years* is the statutory guidance for organisations that work with and support children and young people who have Special Educational Needs or Disabilities (SEND). This document includes essential statutory information, such as the local services available to access, identifying SEND in schools, and the process of Education, Health and Care needs assessments and plans.

The code of practice can be found online here: www.gov.uk/government/uploads/system/uploads/attachment_data/file/398815/SEND_Code_of_Practice_January_2015.pdf.

EHCPs inform the work of all the professionals teaching and providing support for the child and are sometimes coupled with an in-school 'Individual Education Plan' (IEP), which is a special programme written by the school. The EHCP is a legally binding (Statutory) document. It is binding on not only the Local Authority but also on Local Health Services. According to the code of practice, Local Authorities must consult the child and the child's parent or the young person throughout the process of assessment and production of an EHCP.

Support for ADHD

In a recent study, it was shown that almost two-thirds of children with ADHD were taking medication, but less than half had received a behavioural intervention of any kind in the past year (Danielson et al., 2018). Surprisingly about a quarter had received neither medication treatment or behavioural intervention support.

National Institute for Health and Care Excellence Guidelines for ADHD

The National Institute for Health and Care Excellence (NICE) is an independent public body that provides national guidance and advice to improve health and social care in England. The NICE guidance offers evidence-based recommendations developed using the expertise of the National Health Service (NHS) and the wider healthcare community, including healthcare and other professionals, patients, service users and carers, the academic world, and the healthcare industry.

NICE has published a quality standard on ADHD (2013b) that sets out the priority areas for quality improvement in provision for ADHD in health and social care. It can be found here: www.nice.org.uk/guidance/qs39. It has also published an evidence-based clinical guideline that gives detailed guidance on 'Attention-Deficit Hyperactivity Disorder: Diagnosis and Management' (NICE, 2018). It can be found here: www.nice.org.uk/guidance/NG87.

ADHD: Clinical Symptoms

ADHD is commonly characterised as a condition of behavioural inhibition and self-control, rather than a disorder of skills or knowledge. However, the symptoms manifest in the two primary domains of inattention and hyperactivity-impulsivity.

Inattention is mostly the inability to focus on an activity for longer than a few minutes, which results in careless mistakes. The inattention of a person with ADHD results in them finding it hard to carry out instructions, and they may often fail to finish work. They are characterised by forgetfulness or then may misplace things and be easily distracted.

Hyperactivity manifests in subtly different ways, which are just as disabling. The young child with hyperactivity, for example, cannot sit still, fidgets and appears as highly restless, perhaps always wanting to touch things or talking excessively. Children with ADHD are likely to find it extremely hard to play quietly, and they frequently distract others around them. Impulsivity is related to hyperactivity in that it is related to behaviour but may result in a child not thinking before acting or reacting immediately to a situation and not being able to wait for his or her turn. Hyperactivity and impulsivity are highly inter-related and are often considered as a single construct within research studies.

These clinical symptoms are often debilitating for the child with ADHD and left unchecked can lead to problems at home and possible exclusion from school. The problems associated with ADHD are much more extensive than the core symptoms. These may involve conduct problems such as oppositional behaviour, lying, stealing and fighting; academic underachievement; specific learning disabilities; difficulties getting along with peers and teachers; poor family relations at home; inconsistent completion and accuracy of schoolwork; and poor performance on homework, tests and assignments.

Developing Effective Interventions

One of the problems with the currently available research literature on treatment strategies for ADHD is that there is limited information on effective long-term school-based interventions. The 'one-size-fits-all' approach is typical, with the emphasis being on the reduction of disruptive behaviour, rather than improvement in social behaviour or academic skills.

In developing effective interventions, not all strategies fit all children. One strategy is to use a 'Functional Assessment', which focuses on identifying which intervention is most appropriate for each child, the problem and their unique situation. This method of working seeks to identify the contingencies that maintain behaviours and the situations that set the occasion for problem behaviours. The technique uses interviews, direct observation and the strategic manipulation of situations. Using functional assessment techniques increases the chances of interventions being effective.

In developing strategies and interventions, there are several areas to be addressed, for example, the behavioural objectives; the child's strengths and weaknesses; and the additional resources available to address the child's ADHD-related problems. Likewise, it is essential to consider the severity of ADHD-related behaviours; the presence of associated conditions; the response to prior interventions; and the availability of community resources. A child with ADHD needs support across all situations where their problems happen, for example at home, at school, with friends and in the community.

Behavioural and Psychosocial Approaches for ADHD

The symptoms of ADHD have an enormous impact on school functioning. Medication is effective for changing behaviour but not necessarily for improving children's academic performance. The tendency today is to use non-pharmaceutical interventions where they are available, such as parent training, school-based interventions and child interventions, and to use medication only when needed. However, since effective medications became readily available, they have increasingly been used as an effective frontline strategy for reducing the symptoms of ADHD.

Behavioural Management

Many children respond well to the management of their symptoms without medication. Behavioural management involves, "...giving children clear rules, consistently enforced in a calm atmosphere" (Taylor, 2007, p. 155). With this type of non-pharmaceutical intervention, generous praise is given immediately following behaviour that is viewed as desirable, and a clear reward system supports this. This kind of treatment reportedly works well on the secondary symptoms that are often the most troublesome, such as oppositional behaviour and conduct or anti-social behaviour problems. However, behavioural management does not target the core problems of ADHD; for this, the role of appropriately prescribed medications is commonly regarded as most effective.

ADHD affects many aspects of the lives of children and young people. Children and young people with moderate ADHD are often offered a referral to a psychological group treatment programme where the resources of the Local Authority allow this. Psychological treatment programmes aim to improve their daily functioning and their relationships with family members, carers and peers.

NICE gives extensive guidance on psychological treatments for children and young people with ADHD on its website: www.nice.org.uk/guidance/QS39/chapter/Quality-statement-5-Psychological-treatments-for-children-and-young-people.

Psychosocial Interventions

There are a large variety of psychosocial methods used to address the behavioural and social issues that arise in children with ADHD. Behavioural interventions are frequently recommended as ADHD treatments. However, a meta-analysis found no effects directly on the core ADHD symptoms of inattention or hyperactivity-impulsivity when raters were blind to treatment allocation (Daley et al., 2015).

By contrast, a synthesis of findings from top-quality systematic reviews and meta-analyses of ADHD studies revealed that psychosocial treatments contribute to improvements in real-world measures, such as behaviour and social outcomes (Watson, Richels, Michalek, & Raymer, 2015). It seems that psychosocial interventions have a valuable role to play in the improvement of the lives of people with ADHD, if not directly in the underlying core markers.

The NICE quality standard for ADHD (2013b) calls for coordinated services to provide a person-centred, integrated approach to providing services, and this is fundamental to delivering high-quality care for people with ADHD. Behaviour therapies can involve contingency management strategies, parent training in behaviour management methods and teacher training in classroom management. They can also include social skills training (geared towards changing abnormal behaviour) and contingency management using a reward system to reinforce good behaviour and can be given alongside traditional psychotherapy that helps to build up feelings of self-worth. Family therapy can also provide a significant role, where appropriate, to improve the family dynamic.

Parent Training

Parent training is an approach that focuses on parenting skills, the child's behaviour and family relationships. This approach should not imply that parents are to blame for the symptoms of ADHD in their children; rather, that they can be an intrinsic part of the solution to their child's difficulties. Parents learn skills and implement treatment with the child, modifying interventions as necessary. It is usually provided by group-based, weekly sessions with a therapist. Often, these courses last for 8–16 sessions and then contact fades. Continued support and contact are usually provided if necessary where resources allow.

Proper training will provide a programme for maintenance and relapse prevention and will re-establish contact for major developmental transitions (e.g. adolescence). This type of intervention can be offered, for example, in primary care, schools, nurseries or community centres; can be given by individuals with a wide variety of training; and is very cost-effective.

School Interventions

School-based interventions may be given as teacher training in classroom management. Typically, teachers are trained and implement treatment with the child, modifying interventions as necessary. This training focuses on classroom behaviour, academic performance and peer relationships and can be made widely available in schools. It can be given as in-service training and followed-up regularly or provided through a consultant model with initial weekly sessions, then contact fades. Continued support can be given, and contact can last for as long as necessary.

With school-based interventions, there is generally a programme for maintenance and relapse prevention, and this can be given as a school-wide programme that trains all school staff, including administrators. It may also be eventually extended to train parents to implement and monitor.

Child Interventions

Child interventions for ADHD are characterised by behavioural approaches and often focus on teaching academic, recreational and social/behavioural competencies; decreasing aggression; increasing compliance; developing close friendships; improving relationships with adults; and building self-efficacy. They can be implemented by paraprofessionals, which may have cost advantages. These may be intensive treatments such as summer treatment programmes and/or after-school or weekend sessions. These types of interventions can be continued if necessary.

Psychopharmacology (medication) in ADHD

Appropriately prescribed and titrated medications for children with ADHD can allow most to return to normal functioning and help to get their lives back on track. However, although stimulant medications (and other forms) are frequently prescribed for ADHD, their action on the brain is not fully understood. In people with ADHD, they seem to affect the parts of the brain that control attention and regulate behaviour, but their effect is not unique to those with ADHD. These medications work mostly in the same way for all people, even if they do not have ADHD. They help to focus attention and to reduce over-activity and impulsivity. When correctly prescribed, introduced and monitored, stimulant medications, such as Methylphenidate, can lead to a 60–80 percent reduction in acute ADHD symptoms (Barkley, 2004).

NICE (2018) gives extensive guidance on the diagnosis and management of ADHD. Further information can be found on its website here: https://www.nice.org.uk/guidance/NG87.

There are several common medications available for people with ADHD. Methylphenidate (Ritalin®) is the most well-known, but Atomoxetine (Strattera®) and Dexamphetamine (Dexedrine®) have also been also possible choices, as well as many other types of medication. When deciding which to use, doctors are recommended to consider if there are existing conditions such as epilepsy. They are also advised to review the side effects and issues that may prevent the person from taking the medication at a specific time, such as the school day, and the individual preference of the child or adolescent and/or their family or carer (NICE, 2018). Taking these medications typically results in fast but temporary improvements for children in both performance and social interaction.

NICE also cautions that doctors should consider the possibility that the medicine may be misused or passed on to another person for misuse. Treatment should only be started after a specialist has thoroughly assessed the child or adolescent to confirm the diagnosis. Once treatment has been started, it can be continued and monitored by a General Practitioner.

Stimulants are prescribed for about 4 percent of school-age children in the United States, and annual global expenditure on ADHD medications is measured in billions of dollars. The United States, Canada, Australia and the UK are the countries that prescribe the most medications for ADHD, but spending is increasing in both developed and developing countries around the world. The United States is an outlier among developed countries in its high usage rates of these medications among children.

The majority of children and adolescents diagnosed with ADHD in the United States receive stimulant medications or related drugs (Scheffler, Hinshaw, Modrek, & Levine, 2007). Other countries, however, are beginning to follow this trend. The use of ADHD medications in other nations in recent years has increased at rates even higher than those in the United States, and the countries using the most ADHD medications per capita are those with the highest incomes. Given the high prevalence and the increasing use of these drugs, the condition is likely to become the world's leading childhood disorder treated with medication. These findings challenge the widespread belief that ADHD is primarily a United States condition (Scheffler et al., 2007).

Under optimal conditions, stimulant medications can improve sustained attention, response inhibition, persistence with tasks, compliance with instructions, assist academic productivity and accuracy, and rates of skill acquisition. Effective medication treatment can also help to reduce excessive motor activity, disruptive behaviour and rates of aggression. However, the benefits of using stimulant medications must be balanced with the side effects that are reported in some instances. The most frequently reported side effects are appetite reduction, insomnia, irritability, headaches and stomach aches. Less commonly, there can be motor and/or vocal tics. However, the presence of side effects seems to vary across people, and there can be long-term effects of mild weight loss (e.g. a few pounds in the first 1–2 years). One of the main benefits of using medication effectively is a decrease in classroom disruption and the chance to get the child back on track with their education.

However, medication alone is rarely sufficient to bring a child to the normal range of functioning. It works only if the medication is taken and is not effective for all children. It does not affect directly several relevant variables, for example, academic achievement and concurrent family problems. There is also reduced compliance reported in its long-term use, and parents are rarely satisfied with medication alone.

There is an excellent public access article that summarises 'Psychopharmacology: concepts and opinions about the use of stimulant medications' by Swanson and Volkopw (2009) that can be accessed here: https://www.ncbi.nlm.nih.gov/pmc/articles/PMC2681087/

People with ADHD who are starting drug treatment have their initial drug dose adjusted, their response assessed by a specialist and review at least annually to evaluate their need for continued treatment. NICE gives extensive guidance on starting medication on its website: www.nice.org.uk/guidance/QS39/chapter/Quality-statement-6-Starting-drug-treatment.

Other Support for ADHD

Other strategies and treatments are commonly used for ADHD but are not extensively evidence-based, and there are different anecdotal data in support of these approaches. When considering such types of support for children with ADHD one must first seek evidence of their effectiveness and the possible costs involved, both ethically and financially. These are strategies such as traditional one-to-one therapy or counselling; cognitive therapy; elimination diets; biofeedback; neural therapy; attention (EEG) training; allergy treatments; chiropractic treatments; perceptual or motor training; Sensory Integration Training; pet therapy and dietary supplements.

The Multimodal Treatment of ADHD Study

The Multimodal Treatment of Attention-Deficit Hyperactivity Disorder (MTA) study was a well-known large-scale multisite study designed to evaluate the effectiveness of leading treatments for ADHD over time. The study used a randomised clinical trial including psychosocial (behavioural) interventions alone; pharmacological (medical management) alone; and combined psychosocial and pharmacological treatments. Controversially, medical management using stimulant medications alone was found to be significantly more effective than behavioural treatments for the core symptoms of ADHD. Surprisingly, behavioural treatments did not significantly improve outcomes of the core symptoms of ADHD when combined with medical treatment.

Despite the evidence, there is controversy about which treatments should be used for ADHD. Immediately following the MTA study, there was broad agreement among many psychiatric professionals and practitioners that medication is an effective treatment of choice for ADHD. The impact of the MTA study was a huge rise in the subsequent prescription of stimulant medications for ADHD (Swanson & Volkow, 2009).

However, all the groups of children in the MTA study, regardless of the treatment they received, improved dramatically with time. After 36 months, the earlier advantage of having had 14 months of the medication was no longer apparent, "...possibly due to age-related decline in ADHD symptoms, changes in medication management intensity, or starting or stopping medications altogether" (Jensen et al., 2007). Even though their daily dose of stimulant medication had increased significantly, children from the MTA study who were still taking medication 8 years on reportedly showed no better symptom improvement than non-medicated children.

Although the MTA data provided support for the reduction of symptoms with rigorous 'medication management', the long-term follow-up data failed to provide support for long-term advantage of medication treatment (Molina et al., 2009). Decisions about beginning, continuing, and ending medication may have to be made on an individual level.

Controversy Surrounding ADHD

Historically there has been controversy over the classification of ADHD, especially the diagnosis that is established by a review of the symptoms and impairments. Some prominent practitioners and researchers claim that ADHD is actually underdiagnosed in the population (Taylor cited in Banaschewski et al., 2015), while others suggest that ADHD does not exist as a legitimate medical condition and is no more than a cultural construct (Timimi, 2005). Some authors, concerned about the possible over-prescription of stimulant medications such as Methylphenidate and Dextroamphetamine, claim that ADHD is no more than an expression of an extreme of a continuum of normal but troublesome behaviour

However, there is a growing movement for greater accountability and an evidence base for using psychiatric drugs in children and adolescents. In recent years, the ethics of prescribing stimulant medication to children with ADHD has increasingly been called into question.

For more information, see the Council for Evidence-Based Psychiatry (CEP): http://cepuk.org. This organisation exists to communicate evidence of the potentially harmful effects of psychiatric drugs to people and institutions in the UK.

The perception is that there is public anxiety about whether children are unnecessarily treated with stimulant medication; if the diagnosis is made too often; and about the long-term outcomes. Whether this is indeed the case is a long-running debate among both parents and experts in the field. Untangling the complex issues of ethics, treatment and research is a matter of much debate.

It is not surprising that, given the misinformation and 'media spin' often associated with ADHD, parents, practitioners and educators may view the condition with some scepticism. However, increasing numbers of children are being diagnosed with the disorder, and prescriptions for stimulant medications such as Methylphenidate are on the increase.

The so-called 'Ritalin debate' of whether 'to medicate or not to medicate' has existed for decades, and everyone seems to have an opinion on this hot topic, especially the popular press. The concept of ADHD is said to be controversial, but this is mainly due to the media and disagreement on treatment. This argument was brought to the fore some years ago when leading ADHD theorist Russell Barkley gathered together a large international collective of researchers and authorities in the field to challenge some of the misconceptions portrayed in the media about ADHD, to publish the 'International Consensus Statement on ADHD' (2002).

The validity of the ADHD classification, its diagnoses and its possible causes still attract controversy from both the public and the academic community. However, as public understanding increases and scientific studies further define and explore the condition, we are moving closer to a fuller understanding of the causes and expression of this complex condition of childhood.

Support for Autism

Although it is tempting to use the so-called 'medical model' approach to think of autism as a disease and to seek a cure, this is perhaps not the most efficient way to consider the condition. For example, many people think of autism as just a different way that a person's brain processes information – a different cognitive style. With appropriate support and education, many children with the condition can learn and develop. However, it should be noted that many autistics feel that 'treatment' in any form is not required or indeed ethical.

Autism can be thought of as a spectrum condition, meaning that there is usually a range of similar features present. It is important to note that the differences between people due to trait variations (e.g. personality) and state variations (e.g. mood) are of importance to consider in relation to any 'symptom presentation' which might characterise a person's autism. It is impossible to decouple the 'autism' from the person, and this is a common misconception about treatment and 'interventions'.

Early intervention can often reduce the challenges associated with the condition, lessen disruptive behaviour and provide some degree of independence. The most restricting traits seen in people with autism are generally not the core symptoms themselves but reportedly the sensory sensitivities described by people with the condition. Simple accommodations can go a long way in remediating the everyday difficulties faced by individuals on the autism spectrum.

National Institute for Health and Care Excellence Guidelines for Autism

NICE has published a Quality Standard on autism (2014) that sets out the priority areas for quality improvement in provision for autism in health and social care. It can be found here: http://publications.nice.org.uk/autism-qs51.

It has also published three evidence-based clinical guidelines that give detailed guidance on the following:

- *Autism in under 19s: recognition, referral and diagnosis* (NICE, 2011). It can be found here: http://guidance.nice.org.uk/CG128.
- *Autism in adults: diagnosis and management* (NICE, 2012). It can be found here: http://guidance.nice.org.uk/CG142.
- *Autism in under 19s: support and management* (NICE, 2013a). It can be found here: http://guidance.nice.org.uk/CG170.

Behavioural, Psychosocial and Communication Approaches for Autism

Behavioural, psychosocial and communication interventions can help to address the core features of autism. NICE gives extensive guidance on treating the core features of autism using psychosocial interventions on its website here: www.nice.org.uk/guidance/qs51/chapter/Quality-statement-5-Treating-the-core-features-of-autism-psychosocial-interventions.

Applied Behaviour Analysis

Despite autism being caused by neurological abnormalities, one of the most effective behavioural treatments for the condition is thought to be highly structured and intensive. Applied Behaviour Analysis (ABA) encourages positive behaviours and discourages negative behaviours to improve a variety of skills. Although it is not limited to autism, early evidence for the approach showed very high increases in intelligence points for people with autism from this form of long-term intensive treatment (Lovaas, 1987). These results led to an upsurge in interest for behaviour modification treatments for autism.

> "ABA is an approach to changing behaviors that uses procedures based on scientifically established principles of learning. In ABA, the behaviors targeted for change are behaviors that are usually socially important to someone in some way."
>
> (Kearney, 2015, p. 9).

This form of behavioural therapy is typically used with young children that are profoundly affected by autism. It is not appropriate and very rarely used on less profoundly affected diagnosed people or adults. An ABA programme involves intensively monitoring the progress of the intervention, collecting information about the target behaviours and ongoing evaluation of the effectiveness of the intervention. ABA developed from and remains closely linked to classic early psychological research on the principles of learning and behaviour.

A central tenet of ABA is operant conditioning. Behaviours that produce favourable outcomes are selected, and those that produce unfavourable consequences are extinguished. The approach is comprehensive in that it teaches all skills (e.g. sitting, attending, imitating, direction following, language, social skills and self-help skills). It is goal driven in that it focuses on objective measurement and the analysis of behaviour and provides ongoing feedback on progress and setbacks. It has an empirical emphasis in that treatments are based on principles and procedures supported by research.

The ABA approach is characterised by the intensity level, which is anywhere up to 25 to 40 hours per week of one-to-one sessions, for as long as three years – a limitation for many families due to the cost of providing it. Not surprisingly, this approach is rarely offered in its full form by Local Authorities. 'Early Intensive Behavioural Intervention' is another form of ABA used for very young children.

Dietary Modifications for Autism

The gluten-free/casein-free diet (GfCf) is frequently reported to be helpful for some individuals with autism in eliminating many behaviours and digestive problems associated with the condition. It requires the elimination of wheat, dairy, soy and often many other foods and often requires a lifestyle change for the whole family. However, the foods can be expensive and hard to find in some areas. Further research studies are needed to establish the relationship to autism and the efficacy of this approach as a treatment.

Other Support for Autism

Other popular interventions and strategies of support for autism include 'Treatment and Education of Autistic and Related Communication-Handicapped Children' (TEACCH), which uses visual cues to teach skills by breaking information down into small steps; 'Pivotal Response Training', which aims to increase a child's motivation to learn and to initiate communication with others; 'Verbal Behaviour Intervention', which is a form of ABA that teaches verbal skills; and 'Floortime', which aims to meet the child at their developmental level and build on their strengths.

Occupational Therapy (OT) and Speech and Language Therapy (SLT) also have a pivotal role to play in helping people with autism to live as independently as possible and improving communication skills. One popular tool that is integrated into some interventions is the 'Picture Exchange Communication System', which uses picture symbols to teach communication skills and facilitates communication in non-verbal children with autism.

There are many approaches, therapies and interventions for improving the lives of people with autism. The National Autistic Society provides advice and information on strategies for autism: www.autism.org.uk/about/strategies.aspx

Psychopharmacology (medication) in Autism

Although many drugs have been used to treat autism, few medications are effective on any of the core symptoms of the condition. In one study, parents of children with autism provided information on the use of psychotropic medicines, vitamins, supplements and modified diets. Forty-six percent had taken a psychotropic medication; 17 percent had taken food or vitamin supplements; 15 percent were on a modified diet; and 12 percent had some combination of psychotropic medication and alternative treatment (Witwer & Lecavalier, 2005).

Although no medication has been approved to treat autism directly, survey data shows that community practitioners are prescribing a broad range of medication treatments, including, but not limited to, antidepressants, stimulants, antipsychotics, alpha agonists and anticonvulsants (McCracken, 2005). People with autism are generally not prescribed medication to address the core features of autism.

NICE gives guidance about using medication with people with autism on its website here: www.nice.org.uk/guidance/qs51/chapter/Quality-statement-6-Treating-the-core-features-of-autism-medication.

Policy and Legislation for Autism in the UK

The Autism Act (UK)

The Autism Act of 2009 introduced the Adult Autism Strategy, putting new statutory duties on local bodies, with the aim of improving outcomes for adults with autism. It set in stone some of the areas that must be covered by the guidance, such as providing services for diagnosing autism in adults; planning appropriate services for young people with autism as they move from child to adult services, and training staff who provide services to adults with autism.

The Autism Strategy (UK)

In 2010, the UK Government introduced its 'Autism Strategy' to introduce a fundamental improvement to the way in which adults with autism are supported. The strategy emphasised the importance of training, stating that autism awareness training should be available to staff working in health and social care. Importantly, the strategy called for local planning and leadership in the provision of services to gather information locally about the number of adults known to have autism in the area and the number of children approaching adulthood and to enable local partners to predict how need and numbers will change over time.

Likewise, the strategy indicated that diagnosis should lead to a person-centred assessment of the person's needs and should be acknowledged as a catalyst for a carer's assessment. Additionally, an assessment of eligibility for care services cannot be denied on the grounds of the person's intelligence. Practitioners should be able to understand how to adapt their behaviour and communication for a patient with autism. The Department of Health (2015) issues statutory guidance for Local Authorities and NHS organisations to help them to implement the Autism Strategy.

The Children and Families Act (UK)

The Children and Families Act 2014 seeks to improve services for vulnerable children and support strong families. It is critical in reforming legislation for children and young people with Special Educational Needs. The Act of Parliament underpins broader reforms to ensure that all children and young people can succeed, no matter what their backgrounds. The changes to the law give greater protection to vulnerable children and establish a new system to help children with Special Educational Needs and Disabilities, as well as help for parents to balance their work and family life.

'Think Autism': An Update to the Government Adult Autism Strategy (UK)

In 2014, the government published an update to its strategy for autism: 'Think Autism – fulfilling and rewarding lives, the strategy for adults with autism in England: an update'. Think Autism sets out a clear programme that the Department of Health and other Government departments are taking to improve the lives of people with autism, primarily through taking actions that will support Local Authorities, the NHS, other public services and their partners with their local implementation work.

The document can be found here:
www.gov.uk/government/publications/think-autism-an-update-to-the-
government-adult-autism-strategy.

In Conclusion

Families of children with autism and ADHD can benefit from having
contact with other parents who are faced with some of the same issues
as themselves. Parental advocacy groups and charities are vital to
lobbying for better outcomes for individuals with these clinical
conditions. They are often critical to pushing forward the frontiers of
research in critical areas. These groups offer information, hope and
support to parents.

The academic and scientific consensus is that there is no 'cure' for autism
or ADHD, but this wording and perspective are centred in the traditional
Psychiatric medical model of disease, and this may not be the best way
to view these conditions. However, with appropriate strategies and
support, many children with autism can learn and develop. Likewise,
children with ADHD can be greatly assisted with the right interventions
and often helped considerably with appropriately prescribed and
maintained medication strategies.

Early interventions can often reduce the challenges associated with these
conditions, lessen disruptive behaviour and provide some degree of
independence. In most cases, a combination of treatment strategies and
accommodations is highly effective at improving outcomes and quality of
life. People with autism who experience the most-disabling symptoms
usually require lifelong support. Many people across the autism spectrum
lead productive, happy lives and are of great benefit to society. Children
with autism and ADHD can achieve significant, comprehensive and lasting
gains with appropriate interventions and the understanding and support
of the community and those who care for them.

Resources

For more information about autism, visit the National Autistic Society at their website:

www.autism.org.uk.

For more information about ADHD and related conditions, visit the ADHD Foundation at their website:

www.adhdfoundation.org.uk.

The Independent Parental Special Education Advice (IPSEA) charity offer free and independent legally based information, advice and support to help get the right education for children and young people with all kinds of special educational needs (SEN) and disabilities.

www.ipsea.org.uk.

If you would like to consider taking part in research studies about autism and ADHD, please visit www.ASDresearch.org to register your interest.

References

Ahmadi-Kashani, Y., & Hechtman, L. (2014). Antisocial Behavior in Children with ADHD: Clinical Presentation, Epidemiology, Etiology, Prognosis and Treatment Approaches. *Journal of Communications Research, 6*(4), 419–438.

American Psychiatric Association. (2000). *Diagnostic and Statistical Manual of Mental Disorders: DSM-IV-TR.* Washington, DC: Author.

American Psychiatric Association. (2013). *Diagnostic and Statistical Manual of Mental Disorders* (5th ed.). Arlington, VA: American Psychiatric Publishing.

Arnett, A. B., Pennington, B. F., Willcutt, E. G., DeFries, J. C., & Olson, R. K. (2015). Sex differences in ADHD symptom severity. *Journal of Child Psychology and Psychiatry, 56*(6), 632–639. https://doi.org/10.1111/jcpp.12337

Baird, G., & Norbury, C. F. (2015). Social (pragmatic) communication disorders and autism spectrum disorder. *Archives of Disease in Childhood,* archdischild-2014-306944.

https://doi.org/10.1136/archdischild-2014-306944

Banaschewski, T., Zuddas, A., Asherson, P., Buitelaar, J., Coghill, D.,

Danckaerts, M., ... Taylor, E. (2015). *ADHD and Hyperkinetic*

Disorder. OUP Oxford.

Barkley, R. A. (1997a). *ADHD and the Nature of Self-control*. New York:

Guilford Press.

Barkley, R. A. (1997b). Behavioral inhibition, sustained attention, and

executive functions: Constructing a unifying theory of ADHD.

Psychological   Bulletin,   121(1),   65–94.

https://doi.org/10.1037/0033-2909.121.1.65

Barkley, R. A. (2004). Adolescents with Attention-Deficit/Hyperactivity

Disorder: An Overview of Empirically Based Treatments. *Journal*

of Psychiatric Practice, 10(1), 39–56.

Barkley, R. A. (2013). *Taking Charge of ADHD, Third Edition: The*

Complete, Authoritative Guide for Parents. Guilford Press.

Barkley, R. A. (2014). *Attention-Deficit Hyperactivity Disorder: A*

Handbook for Diagnosis and Treatment. Guilford Publications.

Barkley, R. A., Cook, E. H., Diamond, A., Zametkin, A., Thapar, A., Teeter,

A., ... Pelham, W. (2002). International Consensus Statement on

ADHD - January 2002. *Clinical Child and Family Psychology*

Review, 5(2), 89–111.

Baron-Cohen, S. (1989). The Autistic Child's Theory of Mind: a Case of Specific Developmental Delay. *Journal of Child Psychology and Psychiatry, 30*(2), 285–297. https://doi.org/10.1111/j.1469-7610.1989.tb00241.x

Baron-Cohen, S. (2003). *The Essential Difference: Men, Women and the Extreme Male Brain.* London: Penguin/Basic Books.

Baron-Cohen, S., Leslie, A. M., & Frith, U. (1985). Does the autistic child have a "theory of mind"? *Cognition, 21*(1), 37–46. https://doi.org/10.1016/0010-0277(85)90022-8

Baron-Cohen, S., Scott, F. J., Allison, C., Williams, J., Bolton, P., Matthews, F. E., & Brayne, C. (2009). Prevalence of autism-spectrum conditions: UK school-based population study. *The British Journal of Psychiatry, 194*(6), 500–509. https://doi.org/10.1192/bjp.bp.108.059345

Bignell, S., & Cain, K. (2007). Pragmatic aspects of communication and language comprehension in groups of children differentiated by teacher ratings of inattention and hyperactivity. *British Journal of Developmental Psychology, 25*(4), 499–512. https://doi.org/10.1348/026151006X171343

Bishop, D. V. M., & Leonard, L. (2014). *Speech and Language Impairments in Children: Causes, Characteristics, Intervention and Outcome*. Psychology Press.

Blashfield, R. K. (1990). Comorbidity and classification. In J. D. Maser & C. R. Cloninger (Eds.), *Comorbidity of mood and anxiety disorders* (pp. 61–82). Arlington, VA, US: American Psychiatric Association.

Blumberg, S. J., Zablotsky, B., Avila, R. M., Colpe, L. J., Pringle, B. A., & Kogan, M. D. (2015). Diagnosis lost: Differences between children who had and who currently have an autism spectrum disorder diagnosis. *Autism*, 1362361315607724. https://doi.org/10.1177/1362361315607724

Bowler, D. M. (1992). "Theory of Mind" in Asperger's Syndrome. *Journal of Child Psychology and Psychiatry*, *33*(5), 877–893. https://doi.org/10.1111/j.1469-7610.1992.tb01962.x

Brown, T. E. (2009). *ADHD Comorbidities: Handbook for ADHD Complications in Children and Adults*. American Psychiatric Pub.

Buchen, L. (2011). Scientists and autism: When geeks meet. *Nature News*, *479*(7371), 25–27. https://doi.org/10.1038/479025a

Burack, J. A., Charman, T., Yirmiya, N., & Zelazo, P. R. (2001). *The Development of Autism: Perspectives From Theory and Research*.

Routledge.

Cain, K., & Bignell, S. (2014). Reading and listening comprehension and their relation to inattention and hyperactivity. *British Journal of Educational Psychology, 84*(1), 108–124. https://doi.org/10.1111/bjep.12009

Castellanos, F. X., Lee, P. P., Sharp, W., Jeffries, N. O., Greenstein, D. K., Clasen, L. S., ... Rapoport, J. L. (2002). Developmental Trajectories of Brain Volume Abnormalities in Children and Adolescents with Attention-Deficit/Hyperactivity Disorder. *The Journal of the American Medical Association, 288*(14), 1740–1748.

Christensen, D. L., Bilder, D. A., Zahorodny, W., Pettygrove, S., Durkin, M. S., Fitzgerald, R. T., ... Yeargin-Allsopp, M. (2016). Prevalence and Characteristics of Autism Spectrum Disorder Among 4-Year-Old Children in the Autism and Developmental Disabilities Monitoring Network: *Journal of Developmental & Behavioral Pediatrics, 37*(1), 1–8. https://doi.org/10.1097/DBP.0000000000000235

Conners, C. K., Pitkanen, J., & Rzepa, S. R. (2011). Conners Comprehensive Behavior Rating Scale. In J. S. Kreutzer, J. DeLuca, & B. Caplan (Eds.), *Encyclopedia of Clinical Neuropsychology* (pp. 678–680).

Springer New York. https://doi.org/10.1007/978-0-387-79948-3_1536

Cooper, M., Martin, J., Langley, K., Hamshere, M., & Thapar, A. (2013). Autistic traits in children with ADHD index clinical and cognitive problems. *European Child & Adolescent Psychiatry*, *23*(1), 23–34. https://doi.org/10.1007/s00787-013-0398-6

Daley, D., Van der Oord, S., Ferrin, M., Danckaerts, M., Doepfner, M., Cortese, S., & Sonuga-Barke, E. J. S. (2015). The impact of behavioral interventions for children and adolescents with attentiondeficit hyperactivity disorder: a meta-analysis of randomized controlled trials across multiple outcome domains. *Journal of the American Academy of Child and Adolescent Psychiatry*. Retrieved from http://eprints.soton.ac.uk/373939/

Danielson, M. L., Bitsko, R. H., Ghandour, R. M., Holbrook, J. R., Kogan, M. D., & Blumberg, S. J. (2018). Prevalence of Parent-Reported ADHD Diagnosis and Associated Treatment Among U.S. Children and Adolescents, 2016. *Journal of Clinical Child & Adolescent Psychology*, *47*(2), 199–212. https://doi.org/10.1080/15374416.2017.1417860

Department of Health. (2015). *Adult autism strategy: statutory guidance.*

London: Department of Health. Retrieved from https://www.gov.uk/government/publications/adult-autism-strategy-statutory-guidance

Empson, J. (2015). *Atypical Child Development in Context*. Palgrave Macmillan.

First, M. B. (2005). Mutually exclusive versus co-occurring diagnostic categories: the challenge of diagnostic comorbidity. *Psychopathology*, *38*(4), 206–210. https://doi.org/10.1159/000086093

Flory, K., Milich, R., Lynam, D. R., Leukefeld, C., & Clayton, R. (2003). Relation between childhood disruptive behavior disorders and substance use and dependence symptoms in young adulthood: Individuals with symptoms of attention-deficit/hyperactivity disorder are uniquely at risk. *Psychology of Addictive Behaviors*, *17*(2), 151–158. https://doi.org/10.1037/0893-164X.17.2.151

Fried, R., Petty, C., Faraone, S. V., Hyder, L. L., Day, H., & Biederman, J. (2016). Is ADHD a Risk Factor for High School Dropout? A Controlled Study. *Journal of Attention Disorders*, *20*(5), 383–389.

Frith, U. (2003). *Autism: explaining the enigma*. Oxford: Blackwell.

Frith, U., & Snowling, M. (1983). Reading for meaning and reading for sound in autistic and dyslexic children. *British Journal of Developmental Psychology,* *1*(4), 329–342. https://doi.org/10.1111/j.2044-835X.1983.tb00906.x

Ganz, M. L. (2007). The lifetime distribution of the incremental societal costs of autism. *Archives of Pediatrics & Adolescent Medicine,* *161*(4), 343–349. https://doi.org/10.1001/archpedi.161.4.343

Giarelli, E., Wiggins, L. D., Rice, C. E., Levy, S. E., Kirby, R. S., Pinto-Martin, J., & Mandell, D. (2010). Sex differences in the evaluation and diagnosis of autism spectrum disorders among children. *Disability and Health Journal,* *3*(2), 107–116. https://doi.org/10.1016/j.dhjo.2009.07.001

Gillberg, C., & Billstedt, E. (2000). Autism and Asperger syndrome: coexistence with other clinical disorders. *Acta Psychiatrica Scandinavica,* *102*(5), 321–330. https://doi.org/10.1034/j.1600-0447.2000.102005321.x

Goldstein, S., & Ellison, A. T. (2002). *Clinician's Guide to Adult ADHD: Assessment and Intervention.* Academic Press.

Gormley, M. J., DuPaul, G. J., Weyandt, L. L., & Anastopoulos, A. D. (2016). First-Year GPA and Academic Service Use Among College Students With and Without ADHD. *Journal of Attention Disorders,*

1087054715623046.

https://doi.org/10.1177/1087054715623046

Gould, J., & Ashton-Smith, J. (2011). Missed diagnosis or misdiagnosis? Girls and women on the autism spectrum. *Good Autism Practice (GAP), 12*(1), 34–41.

Happé, F. (1994). An advanced test of theory of mind: Understanding of story characters' thoughts and feelings by able autistic, mentally handicapped, and normal children and adults. *Journal of Autism and Developmental Disorders, 24*(2), 129–154. https://doi.org/10.1007/BF02172093

Happé, F. (2013). Weak Central Coherence. In F. R. Volkmar (Ed.), *Encyclopedia of Autism Spectrum Disorders* (pp. 3344–3346). Springer New York. https://doi.org/10.1007/978-1-4419-1698-3_1744

Harpin, V., Mazzone, L., Raynaud, J. P., Kahle, J., & Hodgkins, P. (2016). Long-Term Outcomes of ADHD A Systematic Review of Self-Esteem and Social Function. *Journal of Attention Disorders, 20*(4), 295–305. https://doi.org/10.1177/1087054713486516

Hill, E. L., & Frith, U. (2003). Understanding autism: insights from mind and brain. *Philosophical Transactions of the Royal Society of*

London, B: Biological Sciences, *358*(1430), 281–289. https://doi.org/10.1098/rstb.2002.1209

Howlin, P., & Asgharian, A. (1999). The diagnosis of autism and Asperger syndrome: findings from a survey of 770 families. *Developmental Medicine & Child Neurology*, (12), 834–839.

Hughes, C., & Russell, J. (1993). Autistic children's difficulty with mental disengagement from an object: Its implications for theories of autism. *Developmental Psychology*, *29*(3), 498–510. https://doi.org/10.1037/0012-1649.29.3.498

Hughes, C., Russell, J., & Robbins, T. W. (1994). Evidence for executive dysfunction in autism. *Neuropsychologia*, *32*(4), 477–492. https://doi.org/10.1016/0028-3932(94)90092-2

Jensen, P. S., Arnold, L. E., Swanson, J. M., Vitiello, B., Abikoff, H. B., Greenhill, L. L., … Hur, K. (2007). 3-Year Follow-up of the NIMH MTA Study. *Journal of the American Academy of Child & Adolescent Psychiatry*, *46*(8), 989–1002. https://doi.org/10.1097/CHI.0b013e3180686d48

Jensen, P. S., Hinshaw, S. P., Kraemer, H. C., Lenora, N., Newcorn, J. H., Abikoff, H. B., … Vitiello, B. (2001). ADHD Comorbidity Findings From the MTA Study: Comparing Comorbid Subgroups. *Journal of* the *American Academy of Child & Adolescent Psychiatry, 40*(2),

147–158. https://doi.org/10.1097/00004583-200102000-00009

Jones, K., Daley, D., Hutchings, J., Bywater, T., & Eames, C. (2007). Efficacy

of the Incredible Years Basic parent training programme as an

early intervention for children with conduct problems and ADHD.

Child: Care, Health and Development, 33(6), 749–756.

https://doi.org/10.1111/j.1365-2214.2007.00747.x

Kanduri, C., Kantojärvi, K., Salo, P. M., Vanhala, R., Buck, G., Blancher, C.,

… Järvelä, I. (2016). The landscape of copy number variations in

Finnish families with autism spectrum disorders. *Autism*

Research, 9(1), 9–16. https://doi.org/10.1002/aur.1502

Kanner, L. (1949). Problems of nosology and psychodynamics of early

infantile autism. *The American Journal of Orthopsychiatry, 19*(3),

416–426.

Kapp, S. K., Gillespie-Lynch, K., Sherman, L. E., & Hutman, T. (2013).

Deficit, difference, or both? Autism and neurodiversity.

Developmental Psychology, 49(1), 59–71.

https://doi.org/10.1037/a0028353

Kearney, A. J. (2015). *Understanding Applied Behavior Analysis, Second*

Edition: An Introduction to ABA for Parents, Teachers, and other

Professionals. Jessica Kingsley Publishers.

Kennedy, D. (2009). *The ADHD-Autism Connection: A Step Toward More Accurate Diagnoses and Effective Treatments*. Colorado Spings, Colorado: Crown Publishing Group.

Kessler, R. C., Adler, L., Barkley, R. A., Biederman, J., Conners, C. K., Demler, O., ... Zaslavsky, A. M. (2006). The Prevalence and Correlates of Adult ADHD in the United States: Results From the National Comorbidity Survey Replication. *American Journal of Psychiatry*, *163*(4), 716–723. https://doi.org/10.1176/ajp.2006.163.4.716

Kim, Y. S., Leventhal, B. L., Koh, Y.-J., Fombonne, E., Laska, E., Lim, E.-C., ... Grinker, R. R. (2011). Prevalence of Autism Spectrum Disorders in a Total Population Sample. *American Journal of Psychiatry*, *168*(9), 904–912. https://doi.org/10.1176/appi.ajp.2011.10101532

Loke, Y. J., Hannan, A. J., & Craig, J. M. (2015). The Role of Epigenetic Change in Autism Spectrum Disorders. *Frontiers in Neurology, 6*, 107. https://doi.org/10.3389/fneur.2015.00107

Lopez, M. F., Compton, W. M., Grant, B. F., & Breiling, J. P. (2007). Dimensional approaches in diagnostic classification: a critical appraisal. *International Journal of Methods in Psychiatric Research, 16*(S1), S6–S7. https://doi.org/10.1002/mpr.213

Lord, C., Rutter, M., & Le Couteur, A. (1994). Autism Diagnostic Interview-Revised: A revised version of a diagnostic interview for caregivers of individuals with possible pervasive developmental disorders. *Journal of Autism and Developmental Disorders, 24*(5), 659–685. https://doi.org/10.1007/BF02172145

Lord, C., Schopler, E., & Revicki, D. (1982). Sex differences in autism. *Journal of Autism and Developmental Disorders, 12*(4), 317–330. https://doi.org/10.1007/BF01538320

Lovaas, I. (1987). Behavioral treatment and normal educational and intellectual functioning in young autistic children. *Journal of Consulting and Clinical Psychology, 55*(1), 3–9. https://doi.org/10.1037/0022-006X.55.1.3

Maenner, M. J., Rice, C. E., Arneson, C. L., Cunniff, C., Schieve, L. A., Carpenter, L. A., ... Durkin, M. S. (2014). Potential Impact of DSM-5 Criteria on Autism Spectrum Disorder Prevalence Estimates. *JAMA Psychiatry, 71*(3), 292. https://doi.org/10.1001/jamapsychiatry.2013.3893

Martin, I., & McDonald, S. (2003). Weak coherence, no theory of mind, or executive dysfunction? Solving the puzzle of pragmatic language disorders. *Brain and Language*, *85*(3), 451–466. https://doi.org/10.1016/S0093-934X(03)00070-1

Marton, I., Wiener, J., Rogers, M., & Moore, C. (2015). Friendship Characteristics of Children With ADHD. *Journal of Attention Disorders*, *19*(10), 872–881. https://doi.org/10.1177/1087054712458971

McCracken, J. T. (2005). Safety Issues With Drug Therapies for Autism Spectrum Disorders. *The Journal of Clinical Psychiatry*, *66*(suppl 10), 32–37.

McManus, S., Meltzer, H., Brugha, T. S., Bebbington, P. E., & Jenkins, R. (2009). *Adult Psychiatric Morbidity in England, 2007: Results of a Household Survey*. The NHS Information Centre for Health and Social Care. Retrieved from http://discovery.ucl.ac.uk/164862/

Mehler, M. F., & Purpura, D. P. (2009). Autism, fever, epigenetics and the locus coeruleus. *Brain Research Reviews*, *59*(2), 388–392. https://doi.org/10.1016/j.brainresrev.2008.11.001

Moffitt, T. E., Houts, R., Asherson, P., Belsky, D. W., Corcoran, D. L., Hammerle, M., … Caspi, A. (2015). Is Adult ADHD a Childhood-Onset Neurodevelopmental Disorder? Evidence From a Four-

Decade Longitudinal Cohort Study. *American Journal of Psychiatry*, *172*(10), 967–977. https://doi.org/10.1176/appi.ajp.2015.14101266

Moldin, S. O., & Rubenstein, J. L. R. (2006). *Understanding Autism: From Basic Neuroscience to Treatment*. CRC Press.

Molina, B. S. G., Hinshaw, S. P., Swanson, J. M., Arnold, L. E., Vitiello, B., Jensen, P. S., … Houck, P. R. (2009). The MTA at 8 Years: Prospective Follow-Up of Children Treated for Combined Type ADHD in a Multisite Study. *Journal of the American Academy of Child and Adolescent Psychiatry*, *48*(5), 484–500. https://doi.org/10.1097/CHI.0b013e31819c23d0

National Institute for Health and Care Excellence. (2011). *CG128 Autism: Autism in under 19s: recognition, referral and diagnosis*. London: NICE. Retrieved from https://www.nice.org.uk/guidance/cg128

National Institute for Health and Care Excellence. (2012). *CG142 Autism in adults: diagnosis and management*. London: NICE. Retrieved from https://www.nice.org.uk/Guidance/CG142

National Institute for Health and Care Excellence. (2013a). *CG170 Autism in under 19s: support and management*. London: NICE. Retrieved from https://www.nice.org.uk/Guidance/CG170

National Institute for Health and Care Excellence. (2013b). *QS39 Attention deficit hyperactivity disorder*. London: NICE. Retrieved from https://www.nice.org.uk/guidance/qs39

National Institute for Health and Care Excellence. (2014). *QS51 Autism Quality Standard*. London: NICE. Retrieved from https://www.nice.org.uk/guidance/qs51

National Institute for Health and Care Excellence. (2018). *NG87 Attention deficit hyperactivity disorder: diagnosis and management*. London: NICE. Retrieved from https://www.nice.org.uk/guidance/NG87

Ozonoff, S., Pennington, B. F., & Rogers, S. J. (1991). Executive Function Deficits in High-Functioning Autistic Individuals: Relationship to Theory of Mind. *Journal of Child Psychology and Psychiatry, 32*(7), 1081–1105. https://doi.org/10.1111/j.1469-7610.1991.tb00351.x

Perner, J., Frith, U., Leslie, A. M., & Leekam, S. R. (1989). Exploration of the Autistic Child's Theory of Mind: Knowledge, Belief, and Communication. *Child Development, 60*(3), 689–700. https://doi.org/10.2307/1130734

Polanczyk, G. V., Willcutt, E. G., Salum, G. A., Kieling, C., & Rohde, L. A.

(2014). ADHD prevalence estimates across three decades: an updated systematic review and meta-regression analysis. *International Journal of Epidemiology*, *43*(2), 434–442. https://doi.org/10.1093/ije/dyt261

Rafalovich, A. (2005). Exploring clinician uncertainty in the diagnosis and treatment of attention deficit hyperactivity disorder. *Sociology of Health & Illness*, *27*(3), 305–323. https://doi.org/10.1111/j.1467-9566.2005.00444.x

Rajendran, G., & Mitchell, P. (2007). Cognitive theories of autism. *Developmental Review*, *27*(2), 224–260.

Russell, G., Rodgers, L. R., Ukoumunne, O. C., & Ford, T. (2014). Prevalence of Parent-Reported ASD and ADHD in the UK: Findings from the Millennium Cohort Study. *Journal of Autism and Developmental Disorders*, *44*(1), 31–40. https://doi.org/10.1007/s10803-013-1849-0

Rutherford, M., McKenzie, K., Johnson, T., Catchpole, C., O'Hare, A., McClure, I., … Murray, A. (2016). Gender ratio in a clinical population sample, age of diagnosis and duration of assessment in children and adults with autism spectrum disorder. *Autism*, *20*(5), 628–634. https://doi.org/10.1177/1362361315617879

Rutter, M. (1978). Diagnosis and definition of childhood autism. *Journal of Autism and Childhood Schizophrenia*, *8*(2), 139–161. https://doi.org/10.1007/BF01537863

Scheffler, R. M., Hinshaw, S. P., Modrek, S., & Levine, P. (2007). The Global Market For ADHD Medications. *Health Affairs*, *26*(2), 450–457. https://doi.org/10.1377/hlthaff.26.2.450

Slade, T., & Andrews, G. (2002). Exclusion criteria in the diagnostic classifications of DSM-IV and ICD-10: revisiting the co-occurrence of psychiatric syndromes. *Psychological Medicine*, *32*(7), 1203–1211.

Swanson, J. M., & Volkow, N. D. (2009). Psychopharmacology: concepts and opinions about the use of stimulant medications. *Journal of Child Psychology and Psychiatry, and Allied Disciplines*, *50*(1–2), 180–193. https://doi.org/10.1111/j.1469-7610.2008.02062.x

Swanson, J., Oosterlaan, J., Murias, M., Schuck, S., Flodman, P., Spence, M. A., ... Posner, M. I. (2000). Attention Deficit/Hyperactivity Disorder Children with a 7-Repeat Allele of the Dopamine Receptor D4 Gene Have Extreme Behavior but Normal Performance on Critical Neuropsychological Tests of Attention. *Proceedings of the National Academy of Sciences of the United*

States of America, 97(9), 4754–4759.

Taylor, E. (2011). Antecedents of ADHD: a historical account of diagnostic concepts. *ADHD Attention Deficit and Hyperactivity Disorders, 3*(2), 69–75. https://doi.org/10.1007/s12402-010-0051-x

Taylor, E. A. (2007). *People with Hyperactivity: Understanding and Managing Their Problems*. Wiley.

Thapar, A., Cooper, M., Eyre, O., & Langley, K. (2013). Practitioner Review: What have we learnt about the causes of ADHD? *Journal of Child Psychology and Psychiatry, 54*(1), 3–16. https://doi.org/10.1111/j.1469-7610.2012.02611.x

Timimi, S. (2005). *Naughty Boys: Anti-Social Behaviour, ADHD and the Role of Culture*. Palgrave Macmillan.

Timimi, S., & Taylor, E. (2004). ADHD is best understood as a cultural construct. *The British Journal of Psychiatry, 184*(1), 8–9. https://doi.org/10.1192/bjp.JaninDeb

Tomblin, J. B., & Mueller, K. L. (2012). How Can the Comorbidity with ADHD Aid Understanding of Language and Speech Disorders? *Topics in Language Disorders, 32*(3), 198–206. https://doi.org/10.1097/TLD.0b013e318261c264

Warren, Z., McPheeters, M. L., Sathe, N., Foss-Feig, J. H., Glasser, A., &

Veenstra-VanderWeele, J. (2011). A Systematic Review of Early

Intensive Intervention for Autism Spectrum Disorders. *Pediatrics*,

127(5), 1303–1311. https://doi.org/10.1542/peds.2011-0426

Watson, S. M. R., Richels, C., Michalek, A. P., & Raymer, A. (2015).

Psychosocial Treatments for ADHD A Systematic Appraisal of the

Evidence. *Journal of Attention Disorders*, *19*(1), 3–10.

https://doi.org/10.1177/1087054712447857

Webb, S. J., Jones, E. J. H., Kelly, J., & Dawson, G. (2014). The motivation

for very early intervention for infants at high risk for autism

spectrum disorders. *International Journal of Speech-Language

Pathology*, *16*(1), 36–42.

https://doi.org/10.3109/17549507.2013.861018

Wilens, T. E., Adamson, J., Sgambati, S., Whitley, J., Santry, A.,

Monuteaux, M. C., & Biederman, J. (2007). Do Individuals with

ADHD Self-Medicate with Cigarettes and Substances of Abuse?

Results from a Controlled Family Study of ADHD. *American

Journal on Addictions*, *16*(sup1), 14–23.

https://doi.org/10.1080/10550490601082742

Wilens, T. E., & Spencer, T. J. (2010). Understanding Attention-

Deficit/Hyperactivity Disorder From Childhood to Adulthood.

Postgraduate   Medicine,   *122*(5),   97–109.

https://doi.org/10.3810/pgm.2010.09.2206

Willcutt, E. G. (2012). The Prevalence of DSM-IV Attention-

Deficit/Hyperactivity Disorder: A Meta-Analytic Review.

Neurotherapeutics,   *9*(3),   490–499.

https://doi.org/10.1007/s13311-012-0135-8

Wimmer, H., & Perner, J. (1983). Beliefs about beliefs: Representation

and constraining function of wrong beliefs in young children's

understanding of deception. *Cognition*, *13*(1), 103–128.

https://doi.org/10.1016/0010-0277(83)90004-5

Wing, L., & Gould, J. (1979). Severe impairments of social interaction and

associated abnormalities in children: Epidemiology and

classification. *Journal of Autism and Developmental Disorders*,

9(1), 11–29. https://doi.org/10.1007/BF01531288

Witwer, A., & Lecavalier, L. (2005). Treatment Incidence and Patterns in

Children and Adolescents with Autism Spectrum Disorders.

Journal of Child and Adolescent Psychopharmacology, *15*(4),

671–681. https://doi.org/10.1089/cap.2005.15.671

World Autism Awareness Week - Hansard Online. (n.d.). Retrieved 3 April

2018, from https://hansard.parliament.uk/Commons/2016-04-

28/debates/16042848000001/WorldAutismAwarenessWeek

World Health Organization. (1992). *The ICD-10 classification of mental and behavioural disorders: Clinical descriptions and diagnostic guidelines.* (5th ed.). Geneva: World Health Organization.

World Health Organization. (1993). *The ICD-10 Classification of Mental and Behavioural Disorders: Diagnostic Criteria for Research.* World Health Organization.

NOTES

Printed in Great Britain
by Amazon